drkamalkv's

AIIMS NORCET

Preparatory Manual

(for Nursing Officer Recruitment Common Eligibility Test)

Volume - 2

Dr. Kamal KV

MBBS, MS (Orthopedics)

Foreign (academic) trips (Countries and cities):

Georgia (Tbilisi, Batumi)

Russia (Nalchik, Cheboksary, Stavropol, Kazan)

Kyrgyzstan (Jalalabad, Osh, Bishkek)

Nepal (Bharatpur, Bhairahawa, Dharan)

Ukraine (Vinnytsia, Kiev)

China (Ningbo, Nanchang, Nanning, Dali, Fuzhou, Guangzhou)

Belarus (Minsk)

Kazakhstan (Almaty)

Uzbekistan (Fergana)

Peepee Publishers and Distributors Private Limited®

AIIMS – NORCET PREPARATORY MANUAL (Volume - 2)

Published by
Pawaninder P. Vij and Anupam Vij
Peepee Publishers and Distributors Private Limited
Head Office: 160, Shakti Vihar, Pitam Pura, Delhi-110 034 (India)

Correspondence Address:
7/31, First Floor, Ansari Road, Daryaganj
New Delhi-110 002 (India)
Ph: 41512412, 9811156083
e-mail: peepee160@yahoo.co.in
e-mail: peepee160@gmail.com
www.peepeepub.com
join us on facebook.com/pp.publishers

First Edition: 2024

ISBN: 978-81-9651-877-6

PREFACE

We all know that the exam pattern of AIIMS-NORCET is upgrading nowadays. Hence, you must have observed that the MCQs, which are being asked nowadays in AIIMS-NORCET, are not always from the conventional MCQ bank. It seems, the exam conducting body is framing MCQs from some other medical level exams like FMGE, NEET-PG etc. Moreover, for an exam of AIIMS standard, your preparation must be a step ahead of others. So, I have compiled a little bit more detailed notes, taking references from medical books, so that your level of preparation is at par with the standard of exam. The notes presented in this book are little detailed, but believe me, it will give an edge above others.

As I always say, students are the best judge of an author's work. In addition, I personally feel, there is always enough room left for further improvement. Therefore, I expect my dear students to share their valuable feedbacks regarding betterment of subsequent editions.

Despite my best efforts, some errors must have crept in. Since I have typed the entire content myself, I expect a few spelling mistakes. I request dear readers, to share the same with me (on the channels mentioned below).

Until now, students had supported all my titles. I hope the same kind of response for this title too.

Errata of this title (if any) would be updated on my **WhatsApp** group.

Please do join this group for other relevant updates as well.

Hope this title will serve its purpose.

drkamalkv

07 March 2024

Contact:

WhatsApp: **84 7000 4333**

Android App: **drkamalkvgroup**

SPECIAL THANKS

I would like to convey my heartfelt thanks to all those, who had arranged or served me during my foreign (academic) trips.

No.	***Countries***	***College***		***First visit***
1	**Georgia**	*i.*	*Tbilisi*	Feb 2018
		ii.	*Batumi*	Feb 2018
2	**Russia**	*iii.*	*Nalchik*	Oct 2018
		iv.	*Cheboksary*	Oct 2018
		v.	*Stavropol*	Mar 2019
		vi.	*Kazan*	Mar 2019
3	**Kyrgyzstan**	*vii.*	*Jalalabad*	Dec 2018
		viii.	*Osh*	May 2019
		ix.	*Bishkek*	Dec 2022
4	**Nepal**	*x.*	*Bhairahawa*	May 2019
		xi.	*Bharatpur*	May 2019
		xii.	*Dharan*	Sep 2019
5	**Ukraine**	*xiii.*	*Vinnytsia*	Nov 2019
		xiv.	*Kiev*	Nov 2019
6	**China**	*xv.*	*Ningbo*	Oct 2018
		xvi.	*Nanchang*	Nov 2018
		xvii.	*Nanning*	Nov 2018
		xviii.	*Dali*	Nov 2018
		xix.	*Fuzhou*	June 2019
		xx.	*Guangzhou*	June 2019
7	**Belarus**	*xxi.*	*Minsk*	Jan 2020
8	**Kazakhstan**	*xxii.*	*Almaty*	April 2023
9	**Uzbekistan**	*xxiii.*	*Fergana*	Feb 2024

drkamalkv

Contact:

WhatsApp: **84 7000 4333**

Facebook: **drkamalkvgroup**

AN IDEAL WAY TO SCORE GOOD IN EXAMINATION

In the following paragraphs, I will sum up some important factors, which should be considered for optimum result.

First crucial factor is 'Time': One has only few months (theoretically) to prepare and so many subjects to cover (considering every subject as a separate one).

Now, even in this period, the initial one month is not used for studies by most of the students.

Freshers may use the initial time for searching the best coaching classes/online app/study matter and so on.

Similarly, after the result, the people who could not make it need some time to overcome the setbacks and prepare themselves again for the exam.

Second important factor is 'What to study'. There are no definitive guidelines regarding the content and the depth of studies.

Since this is an AIIMS level examination, you must literally read everything and that too in detail.

Instead of chasing after many books/app, please choose one (with which you are comfortable) and go through it keeping the time restrictions in mind. The better example is that there are plenty of students, who just read one particular app since beginning, and came up with excellence.

Going through the past years, MCQs bank is of utmost importance for every exam, and for this one too. Needless to say, previous years MCQ bank gives you an idea that which all topics (at least) you need to be perfect with.

Third important factor is 'How to study'. Make sure you cover the syllabus in detail at least once and two revisions (up to this much is practically possible). Anything studied is of no use unless and until it is revised.

When you are going through the things in detail, just mark the important things/confusing things, and revise only these things during the revision phase. Similarly, while reading MCQs, put a cross in front of those MCQs which you can answer very easily (it means you do not need to revise them again).

Revising the matter, which you know very well, is often suicidal. It gives you a false feeling as if you know too much and, secondly and more importantly, consumes a lot of time.

It is not practically possible to revise everything. Therefore, some segregation needs to be done. Starting from day 1 of your preparation, that what all content you have to revise later.

So, give the initial three months for detailed study and revise the important (segregated) things in the subsequent months.

One important factor, please 'be positive' in your approach while preparing. For clearing an examination, you need to have two important things: Self-belief, that yes, I have the potential and I will definitely score well in the exam.

I can sense the amount of psychological pressure on the students, and with such a big burden on your chest, it is very difficult to get rid of this feeling, but still try to overcome this fear.

It will definitely help you in performing well in the examination hall.

Most important factor is 'What is your approach in the examination hall'. You may have prepared well but until and unless you apply your knowledge in examination hall, everything is a sheer waste.

So, enter the examination hall with a positive note. Say to yourself repeatedly, 'I have prepared well and I am going to perform well'.

Lastly, the crucial factor is 'How do you solve the paper'. I advise the students to divide the time slot into three parts. Now let us discuss, what is this **3 phases theory** of solving the paper in the examination hall.

Total duration of the examination can be divided into 3 phases.

In the **first phase**, read all the questions properly. Try to mark out the negative statements, like Except, False, etc. In addition, read the MCQ statements properly and get to know what is asked. Do not be in any haste, as it may lead to errors. Say, for example, the questions may be like this: 'In Wilson's disease, what is being used for management'. A student in haste / panic may not understand the things properly, may presume that the question asks about the substance deposited in Wilson's disease, and will mark the answer as Copper (whereas the right answer is Zinc). In this phase, one should be able to solve the simplest questions (may be around 40–60), which need not much effort. Therefore, in first phase, read all the MCQs and answer the simpler ones (one-liner kind of questions). Avoid solving calculation based, all-except or other questions which demand time and concentration.

The **second phase** are very crucial as in this time slot; you have to read the remaining questions again with concentration. For many questions, you may have to think hard to get up to the proper answer. In this phase, you may come across many questions in which you may be confused between two options. Apply your knowledge to get to the most appropriate answer. This phase should be utilized for solving match the following, multiple correct options, all except kind of questions.

In the **last phase**, simply have a look at the answers you have marked, avoiding the tendency of changing the answers. It is a common observation that most of the times; we replace a right answer with wrong one.

In exams with negative marking, for some questions 'neglect' is a better choice than 'act'. If you don't know anything about the question, it is better you leave that question (unless you are aiming for top 10 rank). Guess work should be applied to only those questions where you can rule out two of the options.

This is my advice. You can modify the plan as per your convenience.

drkamalkv
Contact:
WhatsApp: **84 7000 4333**
You Tube: **drkamalkvgroup**

CONTENTS

CHAPTER 1

Medical and Surgical Nursing

SECTION 1: BASICS OF ANATOMY

I. GENERAL ANATOMY

BONE

Parts of a long bone:

- Diaphysis
- Metaphysis
- Epiphysis

Diaphysis:

- Strongest portion
- Contains Haversian canals
- Also known as shaft

Metaphysis:

- Region of active growth
- Highly vascular area
- Lies between epiphysis and diaphysis

Epiphysis:

- Forms the articular end of a long bone
- Covered by articular cartilage

Epiphyseal growth plate:

- Area of longitudinal bone growth
- Present in children only (not in adults)
- Lies between epiphysis and metaphysis

CARTILAGE

Elastic cartilage:

- Present in ear

Fibrocartilage:

- Knee meniscus
- Intervertebral disc
- Glenoidal and acetabular labrum
- Articular disc

Hyaline cartilage:

- Present on articular surfaces of synovial joints
- Respiratory cartilage (trachea, bronchus, larynx, nasal septum)

II. THORAX

SKELETAL FRAMEWORK OF THORAX

True ribs:

- Articulates directly with sternum through costal cartilages
- 1st to 7th ribs are true ribs

False ribs:

- These ribs do not articulate directly with sternum
- 8th to 12th ribs are false ribs

Floating ribs:

- Anterior ends are free
- 11th and 12th

Thoracic vertebrae:

- 12 in number
- Also written as dorsal vertebra
- Contains articular facet for ribs on vertebral bodies

Muscles of thoracic wall:

- External intercostals
- Internal intercostals/IIC
- Transverse thoracis/TC
- All muscles are supplied by intercostal nerves
- Neurovascular bundle lies between IIC and TT muscles

HEART

Surfaces:

- Base: Formed by left atrium and right atrium
- Apex: Formed by left ventricle
- Inferior surface of the heart is formed by: Both ventricles

Arterial supply of heart:

- Right Coronary artery (Main branches are Posterior Descending and Marginal artery) supplies:
  - o Right atrium and ventricle
  - o Posterior 1/3rd of interventricular septum
  - o SA node (in 60% cases) and AV node
- Left Coronary artery (Main branches are Left Anterior Descending and Circumflex artery) supplies:
  - o Anterior 2/3rd of interventricular septum
  - o SA node (in 40% cases)
  - o Anterior part of right and left ventricle
  - o Lateral wall of left ventricle

THORACIC DUCT

Thoracic duct:

- Thoracic duct crosses from right to left at the level of: T4/T5
- Thoracic duct passes through which opening: Aortic opening of diaphragm
- Thoracic duct is also known as: Pecquets duct

LUNGS

Right lung:

- Weight: 600 gm
- Has 2 fissures: Horizontal and oblique
- Has 3 lobes: Superior, middle and inferior

Left lung:

- Weight: 565 gm
- Only one fissure (oblique)
- Has 2 lobes: Superior and inferior (an additional lingular lobe)
- Contains cardiac notch

Bronchopulmonary segments:

- Anatomic, functional and surgical unit of the lung
- As it is separated from rest of the lungs by a connective tissue septum, it can be separated surgically without affecting other segments
- It has a segmental bronchus, a segmental artery, lymph vessels and autonomic nerves
- There are 10 segments on each side

ESOPHAGUS

Anatomy:

- Esophagus pierces diaphragm at a distance of: 15 inches (from incisor)
- Length of esophagus: 25 cm
- Esophagus commences at: Lower end of cricoids
- Epithelium of esophagus: Stratified squamous non-keratinized

Constrictions of esophagus:

- 15 cm (Cricopharynx)
- 25 cm (Aortic arch)
- 27 cm (Left bronchus)
- 40 cm (Diaphragmatic entry)

Esophagus shown three indentations on radiographic study; from above downwards they are:

- Aortic arch

- Left bronchus
- Left atrium

Blood supply of esophagus:

- Upper third: Inferior thyroid artery
- Middle third: Branches from descending thoracic aorta
- Lower third: Left gastric artery

III. LOWER LIMB

BONES OF LOWER LIMB

Hip bone:

- Ilium
- Ischium
- Pubis

Femur:

- Longest and strongest bone of the body
- In 9th month of intrauterine life, secondary ossification centre appears in lower end
- If fractured, can lead to massive blood loss (around 1.5 L)

Tibia and fibula:

- Bones of leg
- Tibia is medial and fibula is lateral
- Common peroneal nerve winds round the neck of fibula, so all fibular neck fractures should be evaluated for common peroneal nerve injury (foot drop)

Tarsal bones:

- Talus (no muscle attachments)
- Calcaneum (largest)
- Navicular
- Cuboid
- 3 cuneiforms

Metatarsal:

- 5 in number
- Counted from lateral to medial

Phalanges:

- 2 in great toe
- 3 in rest of the toes

KNEE JOINT

Muscles and ligaments of knee joint:

- Extensor of the knee joint: Quadricep femoris
- Posterior dislocation of femur is prevented by: Anterior cruciate ligament
- Posterior dislocation of the tibia is prevented by: Posterior cruciate ligament
- Medial meniscus tears are more common than lateral meniscus because medial meniscus is attached to tibial collateral ligament
- Locking of knee: Vastus medialis
- Unlocking of knee: Popliteus

Bursitis around knee joint:

- Subcutaneous infrapatellar bursa: Clergyman's knee
- Subcutaneous prepatellar bursa: Housemaid's knee

FOOT

Joints of the foot:

- Dorsiflexion and plantarflexion of foot occurs at: Ankle joint
- Inversion and eversion occurs at: Subtalar joint and midtarsal (talocalcaneonavicular and calcaneocuboid) joints
- Inversion is produced by:
  - o Tibialis anterior and tibialis posterior
- Eversion is produced by: Peronei (P. longus, P. brevis and P. tertius)

IV. ABDOMEN AND PELVIS

ABDOMINAL QUADRANTS

Planes of abdomen:

- Two vertical midclavicular planes

- Two horizontal planes:
  - Upper subcostal and
  - Lower transtubercular plane

9 Quadrants:

- Epigastrium
- Right and left hypochondrium
- Umbilical
- Right and left lumbar
- Hypogastrium
- Right and left iliac fossa

ANTERIOR ABDOMINAL WALL

Superficial fascia is divided into:

- Camper's fascia
- Superficial fatty layer

POSTERIOR ABDOMINAL WALL

Contains:

- Lumbar vertebrae
- Intervertebral disc
- Muscles:
  - Psoas major
  - Quadratus lumborum
  - Iliacus etc.

DUODENUM/D

Divided into four parts:

- D1 (superior part): 5 cm
- D2 (descending part): 7.5 cm
- D3 (horizontal part): 10 cm
- D4 (ascending part): 2.5 cm

Brunners gland:

- Main function of these glands is to produce mucus rich alkaline secretion which protects duodenum from gastric acid

LIVER

Anatomy:

- Liver is divided into right and left lobes by the attachment of the peritoneum of the falciform ligament.
- The right lobe is further divided into a quadrate lobe and caudate lobe, by gallbladder, fissure for the ligamentum teres, the inferior vena cava and the fissure for ligamentum venosum

KIDNEY

The renal hilum transmits following structures from front to backwards:

- Renal vein
- Two branches of the renal artery
- Ureter
- Third branch of the renal artery

Renal transplantation:

- Left kidney is selected for transplantation
- Iliac fossa is the preferred site for transplanted kidney

URETER

3 constrictions:

- Where the renal pelvis joins the ureter
- Where it crosses the pelvic brim
- Where it enters the urinary bladder wall

PELVIS AND PERINEUM

Uterus:

- Size: 3 × 2 × 1 inch
- Weight: 30 – 40 gm
- Position: 90 degrees forward with long axis of vagina

Cervix:

- Size: 2.5 cm
- Lining:
  - Ectocervix: Non-keratinized stratified squamous
  - Endocervix: Simple columnar

MALE URETHRA

4 parts:

- Penile
- Bulbar
- Membranous (least dilatable)
- Prostatic (most wide)

PROSTATE

Lobes of prostate:

- Anterior lobe
- Median /middle lobe (enlarged in BPH)
- Posterior lobe (most common site of malignancy)
- Right and left lateral lobes

V. HEAD AND NECK

SKULL BONES

Divided into:

- Cerebral cranium
- Facial cranium

Paired bones of cerebral cranium:

- Parietal
- Temporal

Unpaired bones of cerebral cranium:

- Occipital
- Sphenoid
- Ethmoid
- Frontal

Paired bones of facial cranium:

- Maxilla
- Lacrimal
- Zygomatic
- Palatine
- Nasal
- Inferior nasal concha

Unpaired bones of facial cranium:

- Hyoid
- Mandible
- Vomer

SALIVARY GLANDS

Parotid gland:

- Duct: Stenson's duct
- Opening of duct: Vestibule of mouth, opposite the crown of upper second molar tooth

Submandibular gland:

- Duct: Wharton's duct
- Opening of duct: Floor of mouth, on the summit of the sublingual papilla at the side of frenulum (tongue)

TRACHEA

Anatomy:

- Begins at: Lower border of cricoids cartilage (C6 vertebrae)
- Extent of trachea: C6 to T5
- Bifurcation of trachea: T4/T5
- Length of trachea: 10-12 cm
- Trachea has C shaped tracheal rings, which are posteriorly completed into a ring by trachealis muscle

THYROID GLAND

Anatomy:

- Located in anterior triangle of the neck
- Weight: 20 grams
- Extent: C5 to T1 vertebrae
- Two lobes are connected by isthmus
- Isthmus extends from 2nd to 4th tracheal rings

Cells of thyroid:

- Parafollicular/C cells secrete: Calcitonin
- Follicular cells secrete: T3 and T4

VI. BRAIN AND SPINAL CORD

CEREBRAL HEMISPHERES

Nuclei:

- Nucleus dentatus
- Nucleus emboliformis

- Nucleus globosus
- Nucleus fastigii

MENINGES

3 layers:

- Innermost pia mater
- Arachnoid mater
- Outer dura mater
- Middle arachnoid and inner pia mater together are known as leptomeninges

CRANIAL NERVES

Olfactory:

- Sensory
- Perceives smell

Optic:

- Sensory
- Vision

Oculomotor:

- Motor
- Supplies levator palpebrae superioris, superior rectus, medial rectus, inferior rectus, inferior oblique
- Supplies sphincter pupillae and ciliary muscle with parasymapathetic fibres

Trochlear:

- Motor
- Supplies superior oblique

Trigeminal:

- Mixed
- Supplies sensory fibres to the skin of the scalp, face, mouth, teeth, nasal cavity and paranasal sinuses; supplies motor fibres to the muscles of mastication, tensor veli palatini and tensor tympani

Abducent:

- Motor
- Supplies lateral rectus

Facial:

- Mixed
- Supplies motor fibres to the muscles of face, scalp with auricle, buccinator, platysma, stapedius, stylohyoid and posterior belly of digastric
- Gives sensory supply to anterior 2/3rd of tongue, floor of mouth and the palate
- Gives parasympathetic secretomotor fibres to the submandibular and sublingual salivary glands, lacrimal glands and the glands of the nose and palate

Vestibulocochlear:

- Sensory
- Position and movement of head
- Hearing

Glossopharyngeal:

- Mixed
- Supplies stylopharyngeus muscle
- Supplies parasympathetic secretomotor fibres to the parotid gland, sensory and taste fibres to the posterior third of tongue and pharynx

Vagus:

- Mixed
- Supplies constrictor muscles of pharynx and intrinsic muscles of larynx
- Supplies involuntary muscles of trachea and bronchi, heart, alimentary tract from pharynx to splenic flexure of colon, liver and pancreas
- Afferent fibres from the abdominal structures
- Taste fibres from epiglottis and velleculae

Spinal accessory:

- Motor
- Supplies sternocleidomastoid and trapezius

Hypoglossal:

- Motor
- Supplies muscles of tongue except palatoglossus

CEREBROSPINAL FLUID

CSF:

- It is principally secreted by: Choroid plexus
- Choroid plexus is absent in: Anterior horn of lateral ventricle
- Total volume of CSF: 150 ml
- pH of CSF: 7.33

- Main factor controlling CSF pressure: Rate of CSF absorption
- Neutrophils in CSF: Are normally absent

SPINAL CORD

Level of spinal cord termination:

- In adults: Terminates at the lower end of L1
- In children: Terminates at the lower end of L3

VII. UPPER LIMB

BONES OF UPPER EXTREMITY

Pectoral girdle:

- Clavicle and
- Scapula

Upper limb includes:

- Arm (humerus)
- Forearm (radius and ulna)
- Hand (carpals, metacarpals and phalanges)

CLAVICLE

Peculiarities of clavicle:

- Transmits weight of upper limb to axial skeleton through coracoclavicular ligament
- Only long bone to lie horizontally
- No medullary cavity
- Membranous ossification
- First bone to ossify
- Fractures commonly at junction of medial 2/3rd and lateral 1/3rd
- Most common bone to fracture in body

HUMERUS

Nerves related to humerus:

- Posterior aspect of surgical neck: Axillary nerve
- Radial/spiral groove: Radial nerve
- Posterior aspect of medial epicondyle: Ulnar nerve

CARPALS

Lateral to medial:

- Proximal row: Scaphoid, lunate, triquetral, pisiform
- Distal row: Trapezium, trapezoid, capitate, hamate

Carpal bones:

- Largest carpal bone: Capitate
- Most common carpal bone to dislocate: Lunate
- Most common carpal bone to fracture: Scaphoid

SHOULDER JOINT

Shoulder joint:

- Type: Synovial ball and socket
- Shoulder joint is weakest: Inferiorly (Shoulder joint is most common dislocated inferiorly due to laxity of capsule and absence of the musculotendinous cuff inferiorly)
- Shoulder joint is unstable: As glenoid cavity is shallow
- Most common type of shoulder joint: Antero-inferiorly
- Nerve commonly injured in anterior shoulder dislocation: Axillary nerve
- Luxatio erecta: Inferior dislocation of shoulder joint

Rotator cuff muscles:

- Tendons of 4 muscles blend with the capsule and form the cuff
- Muscles are:
  - o Supraspinatus (superiorly)
  - o Infraspinatus
  - o Teres minor (posteriorly)
  - o Subscapularis (anteriorly)

RADIAL NERVE

Injury in axillary part:

- Loss of elbow extension
- Wrist drop
- Finger drop
- Loss of cutaneous sensations

Injury in fracture shaft of humerus:

- Wrist drop
- Finger drop
- Loss of cutaneous sensations

Injury in forearm:

- Finger drop
- Loss of cutaneous sensations

Injury at wrist:

- Loss of cutaneous sensations

MEDIAN/LABOURER'S NERVE

Injury results in:

- Ape thumb deformity
- Pointing index
- Loss of opposition and thumb abduction

ULNAR/MUSICIAN'S NERVE

Injury results in:

- Partial clawing of hand
- Involving 4th and 5th finger

Clinical tests related to ulnar nerve:

- Book test/Froment sign
- Egawa test
- Card test

VIII. HISTOLOGY

EPITHELIUM

Simple squamous epithelium:

- Endocardium
- Endothelium
- Ansa nephroni

Simple cuboid epithelium:

- Proximal and distal convoluted tubules
- Collecting ducts
- Follicles of thyroid gland

Ciliated simple columnar epithelium:

- Fallopian tube
- Efferent ductile of testis

Simple columnar epithelium with brush border:

- Gallbladder

Stratified squamous, keratinized epithelium:

- Skin
- Duct of sebaceous glands

Stratified squamous, non-keratinized epithelium:

- Tongue
- Esophagus
- Tonsil
- Vagina
- Cornea
- Conjunctiva

Stratified cuboid epithelium:

- Sweat gland
- Pancreas

Stratified columnar epithelium:

- Part of male urethra

Transitional epithelium:

- Renal pelvis till proximal part of urethra (include ureter, urinary bladder)

Pseudocolumnar epithelium:

- Respiratory tract
- Auditory tube
- Vas deferens
- Major portion of urethra in males and females

HISTOLOGICAL FEATURES

Histological features and related structures:

- Intercalated disc is present in: Cardiac muscle
- Nucleus in cardiac muscle: Central
- Reticuloendothelial cells of liver are: Kupffer cells
- Space of Disse and space of Mall are seen in: Liver
- Intrinsic factor (Castle) is secreted by: Parietal/oxyntic cells

- Hassal's corpuscles: Thymus
- PALS/Periarteriolar lymphoid sheath: Spleen
- Brunner's gland: Duodenum
- Peyer's patches: Ileum

IX. EMBRYOLOGY

SPERMATOGENESIS AND OOGENESIS

Sperm:

- Stored in: Epididymis
- Acquires motility in: Epididymis
- Capacitation (acquiring capacity to fertilize ovum) occurs in: Fallopian tube
- Length of mature sperm: 50 – 60 microns

Oogenesis:

- First polar body is released at the time of: Ovulation (some says 24 hours prior to ovulation)
- Second polar body is released at the time of: Fertilization
- Oogonia and germ cell are derived from: Yolk sac
- 1st polar body is formed during: Oogenesis

SECTION 2: BASICS OF PHYSIOLOGY

I. GENERAL PHYSIOLOGY

CELLULAR PHYSIOLOGY

3 major class of molecules:

- Structural fibrous proteins (collagen, elastin, fibrillin)
- Adhesive glycoproteins (fibronectin, laminin)
- Glycans (hyaluronic acid, chondroitin sulfate, heparan sulfate)

Cytoskeletal elements:

- Microtubule (Cilia, flagella, mitotic spindles etc.)
- Actin and myosin (Muscle contraction)

CELL ORAGENELLES AND FUNCTIONS

Agranular endoplasmic reticulum:

- Synthesis of lipids (steroid hormones, membrane phospholipid and cholesterols)
- Site of fatty acid elongation, drug detoxification

Rough ER:

- Synthesis of proteins (secretory/exported, cell membrane) and lysosomal enzymes
- Site of co-transitional modifications of proteins (hydroxylation of proline and lysine during collagen synthesis)
- Initial folding of polypeptide chain proteins into 3D structure

Microtubules:

- Cell shape and motility
- Chediak Higashi syndrome is due to microtubule polymerization defect (impaired phagocytosis)
- Drugs which acts of microtubules: Mebendazole, Colchicine, Thiabendazole

Peroxisomes:

- Contains oxidases,
- Catabolism of H_2O_2

Mitochondria:

- Site of ATP synthesis
- Site of Krebs cycle, beta-oxidation of fatty acids, oxidative phosphorylation and acetyl CoA production

Mitochondrial DNA:

- Double stranded, circular molecule
- Inheritance is strictly maternal

Golgi complex:

- Post-translational modifications of proteins (sulfation, phosphorylation)
- Protein sorting and packaging (Secretory proteins like insulin are packed into clathrin coated vesicles)

BODY FLUIDS

Water:

- 60% of body weight (Intracellular Fluid is 40% and Extracellular Fluid is 20%)
- Rest 40% of body weight is because of organic/inorganic material (18% protein + 15% fat + 7% minerals)

Extracellular fluid:

- ECF is 20% of body weight
- Includes plasma (5% of body weight) and interstitial fluid (15% of body weight)

Body fluids:

- Sodium, chloride and bicarbonate ions are predominant in: ECF
- Intracellular fluid is rich in: Potassium
- Endolymph is rich in: Potassium
- Normal anion gap (cations - anions): 10-12 mmol/L
- Measurement of Total body water: Tritiated water/deuterium oxide
- Measurement of Extracellular fluid volume: Inulin, mannitol, thiocyanates
- Measurement of Plasma volume: Evans blue, RBCs labelled with phosphorous-32/chromium-51

Terms:

- Colloid oncotic/osmotic pressure: Pressure due to plasma colloids (albumin)
- Newtonian fluid: Velocity is constant (water)

NORMAL VALUES

Normal values:

- Normal blood volume: 5-5.5 liters (3 liters plasma + 2 liters of cell volume)
- Total plasma protein in blood is: 6.4-8.3 gm/dl
- Normal albumin: Globulin ratio is: 1.8:1 to 2:1
- Na^+: 135-145 meq/l
- K^+: 3.5-5.5 meq/l
- Ca^{++}: 9-11 meq/l
- pH: 7.35-7.45
- PCO_2: 34-45 mm Hg
- PO_2: 85-100 mm Hg
- HCO_3: 25-28 meq/l
- O_2 saturation: 92-96 percent
- Normal glomerular filtration rate: 125 ml
- Renal blood flow: 1200 ml/min
- Renal threshold for glucose: 180 mg/dl
- Tubular maximum for glucose: 320 mg/min

PROTEINS AND THEIR HALF LIVES

Proteins:

- Albumin: 2-3 weeks
- Transferrin: 1 weeks
- Pre-albumin, retinol binding protein, Fibronectin: 2 days

CELL TRANSPORT

Passive diffusion (simple passive+ facilitated diffusions):

- Transport of a substance along the gradient, energy is not required

Simple passive diffusion:

- There is diffusion along the gradient without the requirement of carrier
- Not rate limiting
- Doesn't follow saturation kinetics

Primary active transport:

- Transport against gradient
- Energy is obtained by breakdown of ATP
- Requires transport protein
- Rate limiting and saturable

Secondary active transport:

- Energy for transport is derived from sodium gradient
- Transport against gradient requires transport protein
- Rate limiting and saturable

II. NERVE AND MUSCLE PHYSIOLOGY

NERVE CONDUCTION

Nerve conduction:

- Nerve impulse begins in axon hillock
- Conduction is faster in myelinated axons
- Impulse conduction is unidirectional as neurotransmitter substance is present in vesicles of presynaptic neurons only

MUSCLE PHYSIOLOGY

Muscles:

- Skeletal muscles: Well developed striations
- Cardiac muscles:
  - o Striations present
  - o Functionally synctial and rhythmically contracts
- Smooth cells:
  - o No striations
  - o Found in hollow viscera and eye

Skeletal muscle fibre:

- Sarcolemma covers muscle fibre
- Muscle fibres composed of myofibrils
- Myofibrils are made up of filaments
- Filaments contains contractile proteins
- Contractile proteins:
  - o Actin
  - o Myosin
  - o Tropomyosin
  - o Troponins (type I, T and C)

Muscle contraction:

- Active sites of actin are covered by: Tropomyosin (Troponin T binds to tropomyosin)
- Essential for muscle contraction: Cellular calcium (Troponin C binds Ca)

Muscle proteins:

- Myosin: Major proteins (60%), binds to actin
- Actin: F-actin has an active site
- Tropomyosin: Covers the actin binding sites

Troponins:

- Troponin T: Binds to tropomyosin
- Troponin I: Inhibits myosin and actin interaction
- Troponin C: Binds calcium

NERVE FIBRES

Nerve fibres and their susceptibility:

- Order of susceptibility of nerve fibres to local anaesthesia/cocaine: Type C > type B > type A
- Order of susceptibility of nerve fibres to pressure: Type A > type B > type C
- Order of Susceptibility of nerve fibres to hypoxia: B > A > C

III. CENTRAL NERVOUS SYSTEM

EEG AND SLEEP

REM sleep:

- Occupies 20-30% of sleeping period
- Associated with rapid conjugate movements of the eyeballs
- Though the eyeballs move, but the sleep is deep so it is called paradoxical sleep
- Dreaming/nightmare occurs

LIMBIC SYSTEM

Functions of limbic system:

- Olfaction
- Regulation of endocrine glands
- Regulation of autonomic functions (heart rate, blood pressure, body temperature)
- Regulation of food intake
- Control of circadian rhythm
- Emotions and memory (Papez circuit)

HYPOTHALAMUS

Regulation of water balance by hypothalamus by 2 mechanisms:

- Thirst mechanism
- ADH mechanism

Thirst centre:

- Thirst center is in the lateral nucleus of hypothalmus
- There are some osmoreceptors in the areas adjacent to this which are stimulated by increase in osmolality
- Osmolality is inverse to ECF volume
- When the ECF volume decreases, the osmolality increases
- This stimulates the supraoptic nuclei also, which secretes ADH
- Nuclei of hypothalamus controlling water balance: Supraoptic nucleus
- ADH causes retention of water by facultative reabsorption in the renal tubules

Circadian/diurnal rhythm:

- It is regular recurrence of physiological processes or activities, which occurs in cycle of 24 hours
- Suprachiasmatic nuclei plays an important role in setting the biological clock by its connection with retina
- Nuclei of hypothalamus controlling circadian rhythm: Suprachiasmatic nucleus

Heat gain/production center:

- Situated in posterior hypothalamus
- Nuclei of hypothalamus controlling shivering: Posterior hypothalamus
- Stimulation of this nuclei causes shivering by stimulating primary motor center
- Removal of this nuclei causes a fall in body temperature

Other nuclei of hypothalamus:

- Lateral nucles: Feeding centre
- Ventromedial nucleus: Satiety centre

Thyroxine:

- Hormone important for cold adaptation
- Thyroid hormone increases the heat production in the body by accelerating various cellular metabolic processes and increasing BMR

NEUROTRANSMITTERS

Excitatory neurotransmitter in CNS:

- Glutamate (main)
- Ach
- NO
- Histamine
- Aspartate

Flight or fight response:

- Increased heart rate
- Increased BP
- Increased total peripheral resistance

CEREBELLUM

Comparator function:

- Cerebellum receives information from cerebral cortex and feedback information (proprioception) from muscles
- By receiving the messages from both the ends, corticocerebellum compares the cortical commands for muscular activity
- Based on impulses from cerebellum, cerebral cortex corrects or modifies the signals to muscles, so that the movements become accurate, precise and smooth

Functions of Vestibulocerebellum:

- Regulates tone, posture and equilibrium by receiving impulses from vestibular apparatus

Functions of Spinocerebellum:

- Regulates tone, posture and equilibrium by receiving sensory impulses from tactile receptors, proprioceptors, visual receptors and auditory receptors

Functions of Corticocerebellum/Neocerebellum:

- Concerend with the integration and regulation of well-coordinated muscular activities

Effect of cerebellar lesions:

- Disturbance in tone and posture:
  - o Atonia/hypotonia
  - o Pendular jerks
- Disturbance in equilibrium:
  - o Body sways side
  - o Staggering/drunken-like gait
- Disturbance in movements:
  - o Ataxia (lack of coordination of movements)
  - o Asynergia
  - o Asthenia
  - o Dysmetria and past-pointing
  - o Intention tremor
  - o Nystagmus
  - o Dysarthria
  - o Adiadochokinesia

BASAL GANGLIA

Basal ganglia:

- Forms part of extrapyramidal system, which is concerned with motor activities
- Function of basal nuclei/basal ganglia: Programming of movements
- Caudate nucleus and lentiform nuclei (corpus striatum) are a part of: Basal ganglia

Components of basal ganglia:

- Corpus striatum (caudate nucleus and lenticular nucleus)
- Substantia nigra
- Subthalamic nucleus of Luys

Functions of basal ganglia:

- Control of muscle tone
- Control of motor activity
- Control of reflex muscular activity (posture)
- Control of automatic associated movements (Facial expressions while talking)
- Role in arousal mechanism

Disorders of basal ganglia:

- Parkinson disease
- Wilson disease
- Chorea (rapid jerky movements)
- Athetosis (rhythmic and twisting movements)
- Huntington chorea

- Hemiballismus (violent involuntary movements on one side)
- Kernicterus

Parkinson disease:

- Tremor (static/resting/drum-beating/pin-rolling movements)
- Slowness of movements (bradykinesia)
- Poverty of movements (statue like, mask-like facies)
- Rigidity (lead-pipe)
- Gait (fetinating)
- Speech problem
- Dementia

CELLS OF NERVOUS SYSTEM

Cells and their functions:

- Macroglia: CNS macrophages
- Astrocytes: Maintain blood-brain barrier. Repair and scar formation
- Oligodendrocytes: Formation of myelin in CNS
- Ependymal cells: Line the ventricular system.

ROUTE OF CSF FLOW

- Choroid plexus → Lateral ventricle →Foramen of Monro → Third ventricle → Aqueduct of Sylvius → Fourth ventricle → Foramina of Luschka and Magendie → Subarachnoid space → Venous outflow

REFLEXES

Reflexes and their root value:

- Ankle: S1, S2
- Knee jerk: L3, 4
- Biceps reflex: C5, 6
- Triceps jerk: C7, 8
- Radial jerk: C6
- Plantar reflex: S1, S2
- Abdominal reflex: T7, T11
- Cremasteric reflex: L1

IV. CARDIOVASCULAR SYSTEM

CIRCULATION

Vessels:

- Resistance vessel: Arteriole
- Exchange vessel: Capillaries (maximum surface area)
- Capacitance vessel: Vein

Blood pressure:

- BP is calculated as: Cardiac output X peripheral resistance
- Small cuff, thick walled vessels and obesity will give a: High BP
- SI unit: kPa
- Korotkoff's sound: Produced by turbulent flow in the brachial artery
- Pulse pressure: SBP – DBP
- Mean arterial pressure: DBP + 1/3 (PP)

Some important terms:

- Ventricular end diastolic volume:
  - o Volume of blood in ventricular cavity at the end of atrial contraction (120 ml)
  - o Determines preload
- Ejection fraction:
  - o Ratio of stroke volume to end diastolic volume (SD/EDV)
  - o 50-70%
- Stroke volume:
  - o Volume of blood ejected with each heart beat (CO/HR)
  - o 70-80 ml
- Cardiac index:
  - o Cardiac output/Body surface area
  - o 3.2 is the normal value

CONDUCTION

Depolarization proceeds from:

- SA node → AV node → Bundle of His → Bundle branches

Order of ventricular depolarization:

- Endocardium surface of Interventricular septum (left to right)
- Ventricle from endocardium to epicardium

- Topmost portion of IV septum, base of heart and the pulmonary conus (last to be depolarized)

ECG

12 conventional ECG leads:

- 6 limb/extremity leads
- 6 chest/precordial leads

6 limb leads:

- 3 standard bipolar leads (I, II, III)
- 3 augmented unipolar leads (aVR, aVL and aVF)

Leads:

- Lead I: Left arm – right arm
- Lead II: Left leg – right arm
- Lead III: Left leg – left arm
- aVR: Right arm
- aVL: Left arm
- aVF: Left leg

6 chest leads:

- V1: 4th intercostal space/ICS (right of sternum)
- V2: 4th ICS (left of sternum)
- V3: Midway between V2 and V4
- V4: Midclavicular line, 5th ICS
- V5: Anterior axillary line (same level as V4)
- V6: Mid-axillary line (same level as V4)

Components:

- P wave
- PR interval
- QRS complex
- QT interval
- T wave
- U wave

ECG (Value and coinciding event):

- P wave (0.08): Atrial depolarization
- PR interval (0.12-0.20 sec): Atrial depolarization and conduction through AV node measured from beginning of QRS complex
- QRS duration (0.08-0.10 sec): Ventricular depolarization and atrial repolarization
- T wave: Ventricular repolarization
- U wave: Slow repolarization of papillary muscles

CARDIAC CYCLE

Phases of cardiac cycle:

- IVC (isovolumetric contraction)
- Systolic ejection
- IVR (isovolumetric relaxation)
- Rapid ventricular filling
- Slow ventricular filling

HEART SOUNDS

1st heart sound/S1:

- Because of closure of AV valves
- ECG: R wave
- JVP: c wave
- Starting of isovolumetric ventricular contraction

2nd heart sound/S2:

- Due to closure of aortic and pulmonary valves
- ECG: End of T wave
- JVP: Beginning of v wave

3rd heart sound/S3:

- Heard during early/first rapid Ventricular filling phase
- Stretching of chordae tendinae/papillary muscle
- ECG: Starting of p wave
- JVP: End of v wave

4th heart sound/S4:

- Atrial contraction/last/rapid filling phase of ventricles
- ECG: p wave
- JVP: a wave

WAVES OF JVP

a wave:

- Due to right Atrial contraction
- Heart sound: Precedes S1

c wave:

- Due to right ventricular contraction, which pushes the tricuspid valve in right atrium
- Heart sound: After S1

v wave:

- Due to right atrial filling

x wave:

- Due to atrial relaxation (chordial pulling of tricuspid ring)
- Precedes S2

y wave:

- Due to opening of tricuspid valve
- After S2

V. GASTROINTESTINAL TRACT

SITE OF ABSORPTION

Site of absorption of:

- Iron: Duodenum and proximal jejunum
- Calcium and folic acid: Jejunum
- Bile salts and Vitamin B_{12}: Terminal ileum

BICARBONATE

Physiology of bicarbonate:

- Secreted by: Mucosal cells of stomach and duodenum
- Action: Neutralization of acid (prevents autodigestion)
- Secretion increased by: Secretin
- Alkaline tide: Bicarbonate is released in exchange for chloride

PEPSIN

Physiology of pepsin:

- Secreted by: Chief cells in body of stomach
- Action: Digestion of proteins
- Secretion increased by: Vagal stimulation and local acid
- Hydrogen ion converts inactive pepsinogen to active pepsin

INTRINSIC FACTOR

Physiology of IF:

- Secreted by: Parietal cells in body of stomach
- Action: Required for absorption of vitamin B_{12} (extrinsic factor)
- In Pernicious anemia, there is autoimmune destruction of parietal cells

GASTRIC ACID

Physiology of HCl:

- Secreted by: Parietal/Oxyntic cells in body of stomach
- Action: Reduces pH of stomach
- Secretion increased by: Gastrin, Acetylcholine and histamine
- Gastrinoma is a gastrin producing tumour resulting in increased gastric acid secretion and ulcer formation

GASTRIN

Physiology of gastrin:

- Secreted by: G cells in antrum of stomach
- Action:
    - o Increases secretion of gastric acid, pepsin and intrinsic factor
    - o Increases gastric motility and emptying
- Secretion increased by: Peptides and amino acids, vagal stimulation
- Gastrinoma/Zollinger Ellison syndrome: Gastrin producing tumour

SECRETIN

Physiology of secretin:

- Secreted by: S cells of duodenum and jejunum
- Action:
    - o Increased pancreatic bicarbonate secretion (neutralization of gastric acid)
    - o Reduces gastric acid and pepsin secretion
- Secretion increased by: Presence of hydrogen ions and fatty acids in duodenum
- Most potent stimulator of secretion of secretin is: Acidic chyme

CHOLECYSTOKININ

Physiology of CCK-PZ:

- Secreted by: J cells of duodenum and jejunum
- Action:
  - o Increased pancreatic enzyme and bicarbonate secretion
  - o Increased gallbladder contraction for bile secretion
- Secretion increased by: Fatty acids, amino acids, peptides

MOTILITY

Gastric motility stimulated by:

- Gastrin
- Acetylcholine
- Distension
- Histamine
- Angiotensin

Gastric motility inhibited by:

- Fatty acids
- Acid in duodenum
- CCK
- Secretin

VI. RESPIRATORY PHYSIOLOGY

SPIROMETRY

Total lung capacity:

- Volume of air contained in the lung at the end of maximal inspiration
- 6 L (male); 4.7 L (female)
- Total lung capacity depends upon: Lung compliance

Vital capacity:

- Amount of air that can be forced out of the lungs after maximal inspiration
- 4.8 L (male); 3.6 L (female)

Tidal volume:

- Amount of air breathed in or out during normal breathing
- 500 ml (male); 390 ml (female)

Inspiratory reserve volume/IRV:

- Air that can be taken in over and above the tidal volume

Expiratory reserve volume/ERV:

- Maximum volume of air that can be expired over and above the tidal volume

Residual volume/RV:

- Volume of air that remains in the lungs after forceful expiration

Inspiratory capacity:

- Maximum volume of air that can be inspired after normal tidal expiration
- IC=IRV+TV

Vital capacity:

- Maximum volume of air that can be expired after deepest possible inspiration
- VC=IRV +TV+ERV
- Total lung capacity: Sum of vital capacity and residual volume

SURFACTANT

Surfactant:

- Pulmonary surfactant is secreted by: Type II pneumocytes
- Surfactant is: DPPC (Dipalmitoyl phosphatidyl choline)
- Surfactant production is accelerated by: Glucocorticoids
- Respiratory distress syndrome is due to: Deficiency of surfactant

CENTRES OF RESPIRATION

Pneumotaxic centre:

- Present in Upper Pons (dorsal)
- Inhibits respiration
- Regulates respiratory volume and respiratory rate

Apneustic centre:

- Present in Lower Pons
- Inhibits respiration
- Produces deep and prolonged inspiratory gasp

Respiratory group/RG:

- Dorsal RG: Inspiratory
- Ventral respiratory group (active during forceful breathing): Expiratory

OXYGEN DISSOCIATION CURVE

Shift to left (oxygen remains bonded to hemoglobin):

- Increased pH
- Decreased temperature
- Fetal hemoglobin

Shift to right (oxygen released):

- Decreased pH
- Increased temperature
- Increased 2,3, DPG

HYPOXIA

Hypoxic/anoxic Hypoxia:

- Low pO_2 of the arterial blood
- Seen in high altitudes

Anemic Hypoxia:

- Arterial pO_2 is normal
- Oxygen carrying capacity of blood is low
- Seen in anemia and carbon monoxide poisoning

Stagnant/ischemic Hypoxia:

- Normal pO_2 and normal O_2 content
- But decreased rate of blood flow to tissues
- Seen in congestive cardiac failure

Histotoxic hypoxia:

- Cells cannot utilize O_2 delivered to them
- Seen in cyanide poisoning

VII. ENDOCRINAL SYSTEM

INSULIN

Insulin Increases:

- Lipogenesis (cholesterol and triglyceride synthesis)
- Protein synthesis
- Glycolysis
- Glycogenesis
- Glucose transport (muscle, adipose tissue)

Physiology of Insulin:

- Insulin is secreted by: Beta cells of pancreas
- Insulin secretion is inhibited by: Epinephrine
- Insulin acts through: Tyrosine kinase activity
- Insulin receptor is a cell membrane receptor, a heterotetrameric glycoprotein made of 2a and 2b subunits linked by disulfide bonds; the b subunit has tyrosine kinase activity

PARATHORMONE

Effect of parathormone (produced by chief cells of parathyroid):

- Stimulates osteoclastic activity (increased bony resorption by osteoclasts)
- Augments reabsorption of calcium in DCT
- Decreased kidney reabsorption of phosphate
- Augments absorption of calcium from the gut

CALCITONIN

Effect of calcitonin (produced by chief cells of thyroid):

- Opposite to that of PTH (antagonist to PTH)
- Lowers serum calcium
- Acts by decreasing osteoclasis (bone resorption)
- Hence human calcitonin is used in Paget's disease and osteoporosis
- Decreases proximal tubular calcium and phosphate reabsorption by direct action on kidney

Hypocalcemia:

- A decrease in concentration of free calcium ions in plasma:
  - o Increased neuromuscular irritability and tetani
  - o Chvostek's sign
- ECG finding of hypocalcemia: Lengthening of the QT interval

ANTERIOR PITUITARY

Anterior pituitary gland/adenophysis:

- Derivative of Rathke's pouch
- Synthesize FSH, LH, ACTH, TSH, GH, prolactin
- Release of hormones is controlled by hypothalamus

POSTERIOR PITUITARY

Posterior pituitary gland/Neurohypophysis:

- Develops from down-growth from the floor of the third ventricle (diencephalon)
- Vasopressin and oxytocin are synthesized in the hypothalamus and shipped to the posterior pituitary

THYROID

Thyroid gland:

- Produces T4 (thyroxine) and T3 (tri-iodo-thyronine)
- T4 is converted to T3 by peripheral tissue
- T3/T4 is bounded by thyroid binding globulin/TBG
- Free hormone is active

Regulation of thyroid hormone secretion:

- TRH (from hypothalamus) stimulates TSH (from anterior pituitary) follicular cells of thyroid

Wolff-Chaikoff effect:

- Large doses of iodides act directly on the thyroid to reduce hormone synthesis (it produce a mild and transient inhibition of organic binding of iodide)

HORMONE RECEPTORS

Cell membrane receptors:

- cAMP pathway: Adrenaline, Calcitonin, Glucagon, TSH, FSH, LH, ACTH, PTH
- IP3-DAG: Vasopressin, Oxytocin
- Tyrosine- kinase: Insulin, Growth hormone

Cytoplasmic receptors:

- Steroids (Glucocorticoids, Mineralocorticoids), Estrogen, Progesterone

Nuclear receptors:

- Thyroxine

ADRENAL CORTEX

Zones and hormone secreted:

- Zona **G**lomerulosa: Aldosterone
- Zona **F**asciculate: Cortisol
- Zona **R**eticularis: Androgens

VIII. EXCRETORY SYSTEM

RENIN

Renin Angiotensin system:

- Renin released by juxtaglomerular apparatus after sensing low BP
- It converts Angiotensinogen (from liver) → Angiotensin I
- Angiotensin I → Angiotensin II by angiotensin converting enzyme (in lung capillaries)

Angiotensin II:

- Powerful vasoconstrictor
- Release of aldosterone from adrenal cortex
- Release of ADH from posterior pituitary
- Overall it causes an increase in intravascular volume → increased BP

Renin:

- Action: Converts angiotensinogen to angiotensin I
- Factors stimulating renin secretion: Low BP, Hyponatremia etc.

PARTS OF KIDNEY AND THEIR FUNCTIONS

Function of proximal convoluted tubules:

- Active reabsorption of all glucose and amino acids and most of the sodium, potassium, amino acids etc.
- Passive reabsorption of urea and water

Function of Loop of Henle:

- Site of counter current multiplier (maximum reabsorption of water → concentration of urine under effect of ADH)

Thin descending limb of loop of Henle:

- Passively reabsorbs water (makes urine hypertonic)

Thick ascending limb of loop of Henle:

- Actively reabsorbs sodium, potassium and chloride (makes urine hypotonic)

Function of distal convoluted tubule:

- Actively reabsorbs sodium and chloride
- Reabsorption of calcium (under effect of parathormone)

Function of collecting tubule and duct:

- Reabsorbs sodium in exchange for secreting potassium or hydrogen (under effect of aldosterone)
- Reabsorption of water (under effect of anti-diuretic hormone)

PROXIMAL CONVOLUTED TUBULE

Reabsorption in PCT:

- Major part of glomerular filtrate is absorbed in: PCT
- Substances completely reabsorbed in PCT: Glucose, K^+, Amino acid
- Substances partially (75-80%) reabsorbed in PCT: Sodium, Chloride Bicarbonate, Water

JUXTAGLOMERULAR APPARATUS

Parts of JGA:

- Juxtaglomerular cells (renin secreting cells in wall of afferent arteriole)
- Macula densa (modified distal convoluted epithelium)
- Granular lacis cells

SECTION 3: BASICS OF PATHOLOGY

I. GENERAL PATHOLOGY

NECROSIS

Fibrinoid necrosis:

- Seen in arteries, arterioles or glomerular capillaries damaged by autoimmune diseases

Fat necrosis:

- Necrosis in adipose tissue
- Induced by lipases
- Acute pancreatitis
- Trauma to adipose tissue of breast

Caseous necrosis:

- Seen in TB, fungal granuloma
- Tissue appears cheesy
- Granular material surrounded by epitheloid cells and multi-nucleated giant cells

Liquefactive necrosis:

- Seen in brain abscess
- Tissue is liquefied because of enzymatic action

Coagulative necrosis:

- Seen in myocardium, kidneys, liver, spleen
- Most common type
- Caused by ischemia/infarct

CELL INJURY

Features of irreversible injury:

- Cell membrane rupture
- Caspases activation
- Pyknosis (nuclear condensation)
- Karyolysis (loss of nuclear chromatin)
- Karyorrhexis (nuclear fragmentation)
- Amorphous densities in mitochondria

Apoptosis:

- Programmed cell death
- Lack of inflammation
- Mitochondria plays an important role
- Seen during embryogenesis
- Hormone dependent involution of endometrium and prostate

HYPER SENSITIVITY REACTIONS

Type IV:

- Delayed hypersensitivity
- Cell mediated reaction
- Mantoux test
- Tuberculoid leprosy
- Contact dermatitis

Type III:

- Immune complex deposition
- Antigen antibody complex activates complement
- Acute serum sickness
- SLE
- Arthus reaction

Type II:

- Cytotoxic cytolytic reaction
- Antibody mediated (IgM, IgG)
- Transfusion reaction
- Erythroblastosis fetalis
- Goodpasture's syndrome
- Myasthenia gravis

Type I:

- Anaphylactic reaction
- Mediated by IgE
- Atopic asthma
- Angioedema
- Allergic rhinitis

GENETICS

Autosomal dominant:

- Defect in structural gene
- One dominant mutant gene (A) is required to express the disease
- Heterozygotes (Aa) manifest the disease
- Offspring of an affected parent have 50% chances of being affected

Autosomal recessive:

- Due to enzyme deficiencies
- To express the disease, individual must be homozygous for the mutant recessive gene (aa)
- Heterozygotes (Aa) are asymptomatic carriers
- Both parents must be heterozygous (Aa) to transmit the disease

X-linked recessive:

- No male to male transmission
- Condition is transmitted by carrier women
- Affected males have normal sons and carrier daughter

X-linked dominant:

- All children of the affected homozygous females are affected
- Females pass the trait to half their sons and half their daughters
- All daughters of the affected males are affected, but none of their sons

IMMUNOGLOBULINS

IgM:

- Made of 5 monomeric Ig subunits
- Maximum molecular weight
- Primary immune response
- Intravascular
- Activates complement via classical pathway

IgG:

- 80% (most abundant)
- Crosses placenta
- Secondary immune response
- Opsonizes bacteria
- Activates complement via classical pathway

IgA:

- Secretory antibody
- Key defense for mucosal surfaces
- Activates complement via alternate pathway

II. CARDIOVASCULAR SYSTEM PATHOLOGY

CARDIAC PATHOLOGY

Rheumatic heart disease:

- Consequence of pharyngeal infection with GABHS (group A beta-hemolytic streptococci)
- Type II hypersensitivity reaction
- Aschoff bodies: Pathognomonic
- MacCallum's plaques (left atrium)
- Antischkow's mycocytes (histiocytes)

Acute endocarditis:

- Large vegetations on previously normal valves
- Most commonly caused by staph aureus
- Onset is rapid

SABE:

- Small vegetations in congenitally abnormal/diseased valve
- Caused by streptococcus viridans (organism of low virulence)
- Insidious in onset
- Sequel of dental procedure

Clinically:

- Mitral valve is most commonly involved
- Tricuspid valve in I/V drug abusers
- Roth spots
- Osler's node
- Janeway lesions
- Splinter hemorrhages

MYOCARDIAL INFARCTION

MI changes:

- 2-3 hours: Waviness of myocardial fibres
- 4-12 hours: Coagulation necrosis, early neutrophilic infiltrate
- 18-24 hours: Continuing coagulation necrosis, pyknosis
- 24-72 hours: Total loss of nuclei and striations, dense neutrophilc infiltrate
- 3-7 days: Macrophage and mononuclear infiltration, fibro-vascular response begins
- 10-21 days: Prominent granulation tissue
- 6 weeks: Fibrosis

III. NERVOUS SYSTEM PATHOLOGY

MENINGITIS

CSF findings in pyogenic meningitis:

- Increased protein
- Decreased sugar Raised: Neutrophils

Features of tubercular meningitis:

- Increased protein
- Decreased sugar
- Increased lymphocytes

CNS TUMOURS

Most common primary brain tumour:

- Adults: Glioma
- Children: Pilocytic astrocytoma

Secondaries:

- Most common brain tumour in adults: Secondaries
- Most common from lung carcinoma
- Malignant melanoma has greatest tendency to metastasize to the brain

Glial tumours:

- Most common type of glial tumours: Astrocytoma
- Other glial tumours: Oligodendroglioma, ependymoma, choroid plexus tumour

BERRY ANEURYSM

Berry aneurysm:

- Associated with Autosomal Dominant Polycystic Kidney Disease/ADPKD, Marfan's syndrome, hypertension
- Occurs at the bifurcation in the Circle of Willis (Most common at bifurcation of the anterior communicating artery)
- Results in hemorrhagic stroke/Subarachnoid hemorrhage

For better preparation and success in AIIMS-NORCET Exam, download **'drkamalkvgroup'** mobile app from Google Playstore.

WhatsApp: +91 84 7000 4333

IV. ABDOMINAL PATHOLOGY

HEPATITIS

Interpretation of serological test of HBV:

- Acute HBV infection: HBsAg and IgM-anti-HBc +
- Chronic HBV infection: HBsAg and IgG-anti-HBc +
- High infectivity: HBeAg +
- Low infectivity: Anti-HBeAg +
- Immunity after vaccination: Anti-HBs +

CIRRHOSIS

Micronodular cirrhosis:

- Nodules < 3 mm
- ICC (Indian childhood cirrhosis)
- Secondary biliary cirrhosis
- Haemochromatosis

Macronodular cirrhosis:

- >3 mm
- Post-necrotic
- Wilson disease

Mixed nodular cirrhosis:

- Alcohol
- Tyrosinemia
- Alpha-1-Anti-Trypsin deficiency

V. GASTROINTESTINAL TRACT PATHOLOGY

GIT PATHOLOGY

Squamous cell esophageal Ca:

- Alcohol
- Smoking
- Chronic achalasia
- Plummer-Vinson syndrome
- Tylosis (palmoplantar hyperkeratosis) etc.

Ca esophagus:

- Worldwide:
  - o Squamous cell Ca is most common
  - o Affects upper $2/3^{rd}$
- In Western world:
  - o Adenocarcinoma is most common
  - o Affects lower $1/3^{rd}$

INFLAMMATORY BOWEL DISEASE

Crohn's disease:

- Distal ileum most commonly involved
- Skip lesions
- Transmural involvement
- Granulomas
- Creeping fat
- ASCA (antiyeast Saccharomyces cerevicae antibody) frequently positive
- X-ray:
  - o Cobblestoning of mucosa
  - o Strictures
  - o String sign and comb sign on barium swallow
- Complications:
  - o Abscess formation,
  - o Fistula
  - o Malabsorption

VI. HAMETOLOGICAL PATHOLOGY

ANEMIA

Sickle cell anemia:

- AR (autosomal recessive)
- HbS (heterozygotes) are protected from malaria
- Normocytic normochromic anemia
- Howell Jolly bodies, target cells
- Cholelithiasis
- Most common feature in children: Bone pain
- Autosplenectomy

Hereditary spherocytosis:

- AD inheritance
- Massive splenomegaly, anemia, gallstones, jaundice
- Raised osmotic fragility
- Splenectomy is done

Aplastic anemia:

- Pancytopenia
- Caused by radiation, drugs, viruses, Fanconi anemia, benzene
- Severe anemia, neutropenia and thrombocytopenia with normal cell morphology
- For mild cases, RBCs and platelet transfusion

LEUKEMIA

CML:

- Middle aged adults are affected

- Chronic phase: Stable for several years
- Blast crisis: Accelerates into CML
- t(9;22) Philadelphia chromosome; BCR-ABL fusion gene
- Weight loss, priapism, splenomegaly, anemia, sternal tenderness, painless lymphadenopathy
- Increased WBC (mainly neutrophils)
- Decreased Leucocyte alkaline phosphatase

Multiple myeloma:

- Monoclonal plasma cell cancer, producing large amount of IgG and IgA
- Back pain
- Hypercalcemia
- Anemia
- Primary amyloidosis
- Punched out osteolytic lesions
- M spike (monoclonal Ig spike) on serum protein electrophoresis
- Bence Jence proteins on urine protein electrophoresis
- Rouleaux formation
- Beta 2 microglobulin (prognosis)

LYMPHOMA

Hodgkin's lymphoma:

- Bimodal distribution
- Associated with EBV
- Single group of nodes (cervical)
- Spreads centrifugally
- Reed Sternberg cells (B cell origin, owl eyes)
- B features (constitutional): Pel Ebstein fever, night sweats, weight loss

Burkitt's lymphoma:

- EBV
- B cell type
- t(8;14)
- Most common in children
- c-myc gene
- Starry sky appearance

VII. EXCRETORY SYSTEM PATHOLOGY

Renomegaly:

- Diabetic nephropathy (finally shrunken kidney)
- Amyloidosis
- Polycystic kidney disease
- Hydronephrosis

Contracted kidney:

- Chronic glomerulonephritis
- Chronic pyelonephritis
- Benign nephrosclerosis
- Myeloma kidney
- Diabetes mellitus

GLOMERULOPATHIES

MCD/Nil deposit disease/lipoid nephrosis:

- Most common cause of nephrotic syndrome in children
- Cause: Idiopathic (Most common), Drugs (Rifampin, NSAIDS)
- T cell mediated altered capillary charge of podocyte integrity
- LM (light microscopy): Normal
- EM (electron microscopy): Loss of foot processes

PSGN/acute diffuse proliferative GN:

- Nephritic syndrome
- RBC casts (most specific)
- Cause: Leprosy, bacterial endocarditis, Post-streptococcal ($2/3^{rd}$ cases)
- Immune complexes trapping
- LM: Diffuse proliferation/endocapillary proliferation
- EM: Subepithelial deposits/humps (lumpy bumpy deposits)
- IFM (Immunofluorescence microscopy): Irregular deposits of IgG + C3

NEPHROTIC SYNDROME

Features:

- Proteinuria (>3.5 gb/1.73 m^2 BSA), hypoalbuminemia (<2.5 g/dL)
- Hyperlipidemia/hypercholesterolemia (>200 mg%)
- Edema (Most common sign)

NEPHRITIC SYNDROME

Features:

- Oliguria
- Hematuria
- Edema
- +/- uremia,
- ARF
- Hypertension

VIII. RESPIRATORY SYSTEM PATHOLOGY

ASTHMA

Types:

- Intrinsic asthma: Aspirin, cold, exercise
- Extrinsic asthma: Type I hypersensitivity reaction

Sputum findings:

- Curschmann's spirals: Whorled mucus plugs
- Charcot-Leyden crystals: Crystalloid debris of eosinophil membranes

Sampter's triad:

- Hypersensitivity to aspirin
- Nasal allergy/polyposis
- Bronchial asthma

CHRONIC BRONCHITIS

Features:

- Blue bloaters
- Persistent cough with sputum production for at least 3 months in at least 2 consecutive years
- Chronic airway irritation
- Mucus hypersecretion
- Mucus gland hypertrophy
- Goblet cell metaplasia
- Reid index (gland/wall) is used for:
  - Chronic bronchitis
  - Normal: 0.44
  - Chronic bronchitis: 0.52

EMPHYSEMA

Features:

- Pink puffer
- Abnormal and permanent dilatation of air spaces distal to the terminal bronchioles
- Excess activity of elastase and protease
- Destruction of alveolar walls

SILICOSIS

Features:

- Can acquire pulmonary TB (silico-TB)
- Chest X-ray shows egg shell calcification and snow storm appearance
- Results because of prolonged inhalation of silica (crystalline quartz)

IX. ENDOCRINE SYSTEM PATHOLOGY

THYROID

Papillary Ca:

- Most common (80%)
- Lymphatic spread (slow and late)
- Best prognosis
- Radiation induced
- May arise in thyroglossal cyst
- Psammoma bodies
- Orphan Anne eyed nuclei
- Euthyroid
- Metastatic cervical node with occult primary
- Age: 42 years
- Female: Male:: 2:1

Medullary Ca thyroid/MTC:

- Uncommon
- Earliest lymphatic spread
- Hematogenous spread also
- Familial MTC are associated with MEN IIA and IIB
- Hyaline amyloid stroma
- Secrete calcitonin

X. INFECTIOUS DISEASES PATHOLOGY

HIV

Hallmark of HIV:

- Profound immunodeficiency
- Quantitative and qualitative deficiency of CD4+ helper or inducer T cells
- CD4+ cells are destroyed by apoptosis
- CD4+ T cell count is the best indicator of the immediate state of the immunologic competence of the patients with HIV infection

AIDS related neoplasm:

- Kaposi sarcoma
- B cell non-Hodgkin's lymphoma
- Primary lymphoma of brain

HIV stages:

- Acute infection
- Seroconversion
- PGL/persistent generalized lymphadenopathy
- ARC/AIDS related complex
- AIDS/acquired immunodeficiency syndrome

SECTION 4: MEDICAL DISORDERS

I. ELECTROLYTE DISORDERS

HYPERKALEMIA

Causes:

- Plasma potassium >5.5 mmol/L
- Seen in renal failure (ARF, CRF)
- Low aldosterone (hypoaldosteronism)
- Drugs: ACE inhibitors, heparin

Features:

- Metabolic acidosis (hyperkalemia decreases net acid excretion by inhibiting renal ammonia genesis and reabsorption of ammonium)

Clinical features:

- Partial depolarization of membranes results in weakness, flaccid paralysis, hypoventilation

ECG:

- Tall and peaked/tenticular T waves (Earliest)
- Prolongation of PR interval
- Prolongation of QRS duration
- Ventricular fibrillation
- Asystole

Management:

- Calcium gluconate
- Insulin with dextrose
- I/V sodium bicarbonate in severe cases

HYPOCALCEMIA

Causes:

- Serum calcium <8.5 mEq/L
- Tumour lysis syndrome
- Acute pancreatitis
- Hypoparathyroidism
- CRF

Clinical features:

- Increased neuromuscular irritability
- Spasm of muscles, laryngeal spasm
- Perioral tingling
- Chvostek's sign Contraction of facial muscles, elicited by light tapping of the facial nerve)
- Trouseau's sign
- Carpopedal spasm
- Hyperactive deep tendon reflexes

ECG changes:

- Prolongation of QT interval

Management:

- Vitamin D/calcitriol
- High oral calcium intake
- I/V calcium gluconate
- Thiazides

II. DISEASES OF RESPIRATORY SYSTEM

Paradoxical breathing:

- Unilateral Diaphragmatic palsy
- Flail chest

SPIROMETRY IN LUNG DISEASES

Obstructive lung disease:

- TLC, FVC, RV: Increased
- FRC, FEV1, FEV1/FVC: Decreased

Restrictive lung disease:

- All decreased except FEV1/FVC (Normal/increased)

RESPIRATORY FAILURE

Type I respiratory failure:

- Hypoxia
- Normo/hypocapnia
- Acute: Asthma, pulmonary edema, pulmonary embolism, pneumonia, pneumothorax, ARDS
- Chronic: Emphysema, Right to left shunts, lung fibrosis

Type II respiratory failure:

- Hypoxia with hypercapnia
- Acute: Acute severe asthma, Acute exacerbation of COPD, flail chest
- Chronic: COPD, kyphoscoliosis, ankylosing spondylitis, myopathies, kyphoscoliosis

Type III:

- Perioperative lung atelectasis

Type IV:

- Hypoperfusion of respiratory muscles in patients with shock

ASTHMA

Definition:

- Inflammatory disease of the small airways, characterized by episodic, reversible bronchial obstruction due to hyper-responsiveness of tracheobronchial tree

Types:

- Intrinsic/Late onset: Triggered by aspirin, cold, exercise
- Extrinsic/Early onset/Atopic: Type I hypersensitivity

Factors precipitating asthma:

- Cold air, dust, emotional stress, exercise, drugs (NSAIDs especially aspirin, beta blockers), allergens (inhaled like dust, ingested like fish)

Pathology:

- Bronchial smooth muscle hypertrophy and hyperplasia
- Hypertrophy of submucosal mucus glands
- Bronchial wall edema
- Infiltration with increased number of eosinophils
- Increased leukotriene levels

Microscopically:

- Curschmann's spirals seen (Whorled mucus plugs)
- Charcot Leyden crystals (Crystalloid debris of eosinophil membrane)

Peak expiratory flow rate:

- Diurnal variation of >15-20% is a defining feature of asthma (morning dip)

Nocturnal asthma:

- Overnight fall of more than 20% in the FEV1 or PEFR

Management of bronchial asthma:

- Drugs used for prevention of asthma:
  - o Cromolyn sodium
  - o Ketotifen
  - o Nedocromil sodium
- Drugs used to reverse bronchospasm:
  - o Beta-adrenergic (LABA)
  - o Anticholinergics
  - o Methylxanthines
  - o Anti-inflammatory
  - o Leukotrienes antagonist
  - o 5-lipoxygenase inhibitor
  - o Anti-IgE (Omalizumab)
- Treatment of infection: Avoidance of allergens and other precipitating factors

EMPHYSEMA

Definition:

- Abnormal and permanent dilatation of air spaces distal to terminal bronchioles

3 types:

- Paraseptal:
  - o Spares proximal
  - o Involves distal acinus
  - o Found near pleura
  - o Results in bullae and blebs which may result in spontaneous pneumothorax
- Panacinar:
  - o Associated with Alpha-1-antitrypsin deficiency
  - o Uniform destruction and dilatation of acinus
  - o Predominant in lower basal zones
- Centriacinar:
  - o Seen in smokers

- o Enlargement of central/proximal part of respiratory unit – the acinus
- o Predominant in upper lobe and apices

Clinical features:

- Dyspnea
- Barrel shaped chest
- Respiratory acidosis
- Pulmonary hypertension
- Cor pulmonale

Chest X-ray findings (emphysema):

- Hypertranslucency
- Widened intercostal spaces
- Tubular heart

Pulmonary function test:

- FEV1 and VC show an obstructive defect
- Reduced FEV1/VC
- Increase in TLC and RV

Treatment:

- Stop smoking
- Long term O_2 therapy
- Administer influenza and pneumococcal vaccine
- Alpha-1-AT, when it is deficient

CHRONIC BRONCHITIS

Definition:

- Persistent cough with production of sputum for at least 3 months in a year for at least 2 consecutive years

Pathology:

- Mucus gland hypertrophy
- Mucus hypersecretion
- Goblet cell metaplasia

Clinical features:

- Cough with sputum production
- Wheezing
- Cyanosis
- Cor pulmonale

Reid's index value:

- 0.52 +/- 0.08

BRONCHIECTASIS

Definition:

- Permanently dilated bronchi (by more than 2 mm), purulent sputum, recurrent infections
- Kartagener's syndrome

Causes:

- Bronchial distension as a result of chronic obstruction and recurrent infection

Most common site:

- Lower lobe
- Left lower lobe because the lower lobe bronchus is longer and narrower
- Involvement of upper lobe is uncommon

Clinical features:

- Persistent, recurrent cough and large quantity of purulent sputum
- Hemoptysis
- Clubbing

Sputum examination:

- Identifying the organism
- 3 layered sputum is seen

Chest X-ray findings:

- Ring shadows
- Tram track sign
- Gloved finger appearance

Non-invasive diagnostic test:

- CT scan

Confirmation of diagnosis is by:

- Bronchography

Treatment:

- Control of infections
- Improved clearance of tracheobronchial secretions
- Bronchodilators

PLEURAL EFFUSION

Mechanism of pleural effusion:

- Elevation of venous pressure

- Decrease in plasma oncotic pressure
- Increase in pleural space oncotic pressure
- Increased capillary permeability
- Obstruction of lymphatics

2 types:

- Transudate:
  - o CCF
  - o Cirrhosis liver
  - o Nephrotic syndrome
- Exudate:
  - o Infectious conditions
  - o Collagen vascular disease
  - o Meig syndrome

Clinical features:

- Pleuritic chest pain
- Dyspnea
- Tracheal and mediastinal shift to opposite side
- Diminished/absent breath sounds
- Stony dull percussion note

Cholesterol in pleural fluid (long standing):

- TB
- Hypothyroidism

Chest X-ray findings:

- Dense uniform opacity in the lower and lateral part of the hemithorax shading off above and medially into translucent lung (Ellis 'S' shaped curve)
- Mediastinal and tracheal shift to opposite side
- Obliteration of costophrenic and costodiaphragmatic angles

Treatment:

- Treat underlying cause
- Pleural aspiration (not more than 1000 mL in one sitting)

PRIMARY PULMONARY TB

Ghon's focus:

- Subpleural focus usually at the lower border of upper lobe or upper border of lower lobe

Ghon's complex:

- Ghon's focus + draining lymph nodes

Remnants of healed initial infection:

- Ghon's lesions (calcified parenchymal nodules)
- Ranke's complex (calcified hilar nodes)

Clinical features:

- Fever
- Loss of appetite
- Cough
- Erythema nodosum
- Phlyctenular conjunctivitis may be associated with primary infection

Miliary TB:

- Produced by acute dissemination of TB bacilli via blood stream resulting in the appearance of discrete nodule shadows about the size of millet seeds (2 mm)

Sputum examination:

- At least thrice
- For AFB by Ziehl-Neelsen technique (if bacilli are numerous) or Auramine-phenol fluorescent test (if bacilli are small in number)
- >50,000 bacilli/mL of sputum is sputum positivity

Other methods:

- Culture and drug sensitivity tests using BACTEC radiometric method
- PCR technology
- ELISA testing for IgG antibodies

Management:

- First line drugs:
  - o Rifampicin
  - o INH
  - o Pyrazinamide
  - o Streptomycin
  - o Ethambutol
- Second line drugs:
  - o Thiacetazone
  - o Capreomycin
  - o PAS
  - o Ethionamide
  - o Kanamycin
  - o Ciprofloxacin
  - o Cycloserine

PRIMARY PULMONARY TB

Location of post-primary pulmonary TB:

- Usually situated in the posterior segment of apical lobes or apical segment of lower lobe (because of high ventilation perfusion ratios)

Simon focus:

- Present in apical or posterior segment of upper lobe
- Seedling of bacilli in this area is favoured by high pO_2 of the region

TUBERCULIN TEST

Procedure:

- 5U of PPD is injected intradermally on flexor aspect of forearm
- Extent of induration is measured after 48-72 hours

Interpretation of tuberculin test:

- 0-4 mm: Negative
- 5-9 mm: Doubtful
- 10 mm or more: Positive
- In HIV infected patients, 5 mm is considered positive

PULMONARY EMBOLISM

Features:

- Most common and earliest manifestation: Dyspnea
- Most common sign is tachypnea

ECG findings:

- S1Q3T3

Signs seen on Chest X-ray:

- Hampton's hump
- Westermark's sign

Plasma D-dimer ELISA level:

- Elevated (> 90%)

Most specific test:

- CT scan

III. DISEASES OF THE CARDIOVASCULAR SYSTEM

PULSE

Pulsus bisferiens (rapid rising and twice beating):

- Mild Aortic stenosis with Severe aortic regurgitation
- HOCM

Dicrotic pulse:

- Has 2 palpable waves
- One in systole and one in diastole
- Seen in dilated cardiomyopathy

Water hammer/collapsing pulse:

- Large bounding pulse
- Aortic regurgitation
- PDA
- Hyperdynamic circulation

Pulsus paradoxus:

- Exaggeration of normal; fall in systolic BP of >10 mm Hg on inspiration
- Lungs:
  - o Asthma (COPD)
  - o Emphysema
- Heart (**CC**):
  - o Constrictive Pericarditis
  - o Cardiac tamponade/pericardial effusion

JUGULAR VENOUS PULSE

Positive waves and events of cardiac cycle:

- 'a' wave is due to: Atrial systole
- 'c' wave is due to: Isometric ventricular contraction phase causing bulging of AV valves into atrium/tricuspid closure

Abnormalities of JVP:

- Large a wave: TS/PS/pulmonary hypertension
- Cannon a wave:
  - o CHB
  - o AV dissociation with ventricular tachycardia
  - o Slow y descent: TS

- Deep x and y descent:
  - o Constrictive pericarditis
  - o Pericardial tamponade

HEART SOUNDS

Soft S1:

- Mitral stenosis (long standing, calcified and rigid)
- Poor conduction of sound through chest wall

2nd heart sound:

- Produced because of closure of Semilunar valves (aortic and pulmonary)
- Sequence of valve closure: A2 followed by P2
- Effect of respiration: Split increases in inspiration as in inspiration blood increases in RV but decreases in LV (reverse in expiration)

Wide split S2:

- Pulmonary stenosis
- RBBB

Reverse splitting of S2:

- Left bundle branch block
- Aortic stenosis

Wide, fixed splitting:

- ASD

S3 is heard in:

- Young people (< 30 years)
- MR
- TR
- Hyperdynamic states

S4 is heard in:

- Hypertension
- HOCM (severe LV hypertrophy)

ECG

Waves and events of cardiac cycle:

- P wave is due to: Atrial depolarization
- PR interval (beginning of P to beginning of R): Conduction through AV node
- QRS complex (End of P-wave and beginning of ST segment): Ventricular depolarization
- Duration of QRS complex: 0.08-0.10 seconds
- QT interval (beginning of Q to end of T): Mechanical contraction of ventricles
- ST segment (end of S to the beginning of T): Isoelectric ventricular contraction
- T wave: Ventricular repolarization

PR interval:

- Measured from: Beginning of P wave to beginning of R wave
- Includes Atrial depolarization and conduction through AV node, Bundle of His and Purkinje fibres
- Represents conduction time through: AV node
- Shortened in: WPW syndrome
- Prolonged in: Acute rheumatic fever

Abnormalities in ECG:

- Tall tented T waves, decreased p wave amplitude, widening of QRS complex: Hyperkalemia
- Prominent U waves, small T waves: Hypokalemia
- Shortening of QT interval: Hypercalcemia
- Widening of QT interval: Hypocalcemia
- Convex elevation of J point/J waves/Osborne waves: Hypothermia
- SIQIIITIII: Pulmonary embolism

CARDIAC ARRHYTHMIAS

Types:

- Atrial tachyarrhythmias
- Supraventricular tachyarrhythmias (QRS complex duration and morphology normal)
- PSVT (Paroxysmal Supraventricular Tachycardia)

Atrial tachyarrhythmias:

- Atrial tachycardia
- Atrial fibrillation
- Atrial flutter

Ventricular tachyarrhythmias:

- Ventricular tachycardia
- Ventricular flutter
- Ventricular fibrillation

PSVT:

- Normal wave is followed by QRS complex, but no P wave because P wave S P wave is merged with QRS complex

- ECG:
  - o P wave absent
  - o R-R interval decreased/constant

Atrial fibrillation:

- Heart rate is >350 beats/minute
- QRS morphology is normal
- R-R interval variable and irregular
- Management of AF:
  - o Control fast ventricular rate by blocking AV node (beta blocker, Calcium channel blocker)
  - o Convert AF into sinus rhythm (DC cardioversion)
  - o Maintenance of sinus rhythm (Amiodarone, Sotalol)

Ventricular tachycardia/VT:

- >3 consecutive ventricular ectopic at HR >100 beats/minute
- Management of VT:
  - o Non-sustained: Treat underlying cause (amiodarone, ibulitide)
  - o Sustained or polymorphic: Treat like ventricular flutter or ventricular fibrillation

Polymorphic VT:

- Also known as Torsade de pointes
- Chiefly due to drugs (terfenadine, sevoflurane) and electrolyte imbalance (hypomagnesemia and hypokalemia)
- ECG:
  - o Prolonged QTc (>460-480 ms)
  - o Resting bradycardia (<60 beats/min)
- Can result in ventricular fibrillation and sudden death

Congenital long QT syndrome:

- Known as Romano Ward syndrome
- It is because of recurrent bouts of rapid polymorphic ventricular tachycardia known as Torsade de pointes.

Ventricular flutter/VF:

- Heart rate >250/min
- Only QRS, no other wave seen on ECG
- DC cardioversion and I/V lignocaine followed by amiodarone maintenance

Ventricular fibrillation:

- Chaotic pattern on ECG
- DC cardioversion and I/V lignocaine followed by amiodarone maintenance

HEART BLOCK

Types:

- SA node block
- AV node block
- Bundle branch block (right and left)

AV block:

- Conduction from atria to ventricles is lost
- Types:
  - o Incomplete AV block:
    - – Partial disturbances in conduction (1st and 2nd degree)
  - o Complete AV block:
    - – Complete loss of conduction between atria and ventricles (3rd degree)
- 2nd degree AV block/intermittent AV block:
  - o All impulses do not reach ventricles
    - – Mobitz type I
    - – Mobitz type II

1st degree AV block:

- All atrial impulses reach the ventricles but PR interval is abnormally prolonged
- Atria: ventricle ratio is 1:1
- Abnormally prolonged PR interval (>0.20 seconds)
- Feature of digitalis toxicity, beta-blockers and calcium channel blocker
- Recall: PR interval (beginning of P to beginning of R) indicates conduction through AV node

Second degree AV block:

- All impulses do not reach ventricles
- Atria: ventricle ratio is 2:1 or 3:1
- Abnormally prolonged PR interval (>0.2 seconds)
- Two types:
  - o Mobitz type I (Wenckebach block)
  - o Mobitz type II

Mobitz type I block:

- Normal QRS, but gradual lengthening of PR interval (Wenckebach phenomenon)
- Seen with digitalis toxicity and beta blockers use

- May be seen transiently in inferior wall MI

Mobitz type II:

- PR interval is normal but QRS widened
- Seen in conduction defects of Bundle of His and Purkinje fibres
- Sudden drop in beat without any PR interval prolongation
- Require pacemaker

Complete/3rd degree heart block:

- Complete loss of conduction between atria and ventricles so ventricles beat at a much slower rate (idioventricular rhythm)
- Stokes Adams syndrome:
  - o If 3rd degree heart block develops suddenly, dizziness and fainting may occur
- Seen in digitalis toxicity or myocardial infarction
- Requires pacemaker

Bundle branch block:

- LBBB: Left ventricle contracts after right ventricle
- RBBB: Right ventricle contracts after left ventricle
- Left anterior hemiblock/fascicular block
- Left posterior hemiblock/fascicular block

RHEUMATIC HEART DISEASE

Features:

- Caused by GABHS (group A beta-hemolytic streptococci)
- Follows pharyngeal infection
- Type II hypersensitivity reaction

Minor criteria:

- Clinical: Arthralgia, fever, previous rheumatic fever, RHD
- Laboratory: Prolonged PR interval on ECG, increased acute phase reactants (ESR, CRP, leucocytes)

Major criteria:

- Subcutaneous nodule
- Erythema marginatum
- Syndenham's chorea
- Carditis
- Migratory polyarthritis

Associated terms:

- Aschoff bodies:
  - o Focal inflammatory nodules
  - o Pathognomonic
- Anitschkow cells/Caterpillar cells (large activated histiocytes)
- Pancarditis
- McCallum patch (Subendocardial collection of Aschoff nodules in left atrium)

MITRAL STENOSIS/MS

Features:

- Most common cause: RHD
- Initially asymptomatic (upto 10 years)
- Later features of heart failure:
  - o Dyspnea on exertion
  - o Orthopnea
  - o Atrial fibrillation: 400 $\pm$ 50 heartbeats/minute)
  - o Hemoptysis
  - o Pulmonary hypertension
  - o Hoarseness of voice (Ortner syndrome)

Auscultatory findings:

- Opening snap after S2
- Rumbling late mid-diastolic murmur, which is best heard at apex
- Loud S1

X-ray of chest:

- Straightening of left border
- Left atrial enlargement
- Double atrial shadow
- Right ventricular hypertrophy

IOC for MS:

- Echocardiography

Treatment:

- Most important differential diagnosis: Left atrial myxoma
- Diuretics (for reducing preload)
- Antiarrhythmics (for atrial fibrillation)
- Balloon valvuloplasty
- Valve replacement
- Mitral valve area incompatible with life: Less than 0.6 cm^2

INFECTIVE ENDOCARDITIS

Most common cause of SABE (Subacute endocarditis):

- Streptococcus viridans (low virulence)
- Smaller vegetations in diseased/congenitally abnormal valves
- Occur after dental surgeries

Most common cause in I/V drug abusers:

- Staph aureus (esp. with acute presentation)

Acute endocarditis:

- Caused by staph aureus (organism of high virulence)
- Onset is rapid
- Valves are normal
- Large vegetations
- Splinter hemorrhages on nail beds are seen
- Management:
  - o Multiple blood cultures
  - o Prolonged antibiotic therapy

Terms related to bacterial endocarditis:

- Oslers nodes: Painful, pea-sized nodules in pulp of fingers/ finger or toe pads (SABE)
- Janeways lesions: Non-tender, small erythematous lesions in soles/palm (ABE)
- Spots in retina: Roth's spot (round white spots on retina surrounded by hemorrhage)

Conditions and sites of vegetations:

- Libman Sacks: Both side of valve leaflets
- NBTE/Marantic endocarditis: Along the line of closure
- RHD/Rheumatic fever: Along the line of closure
- IE/Infective endocarditis: On valve cusps, that extends onto valve cords

IV. DISEASES OF THE HEMATOPOIETIC SYSTEM

MEGALOBLASTIC ANEMIA

Types:

- Vitamin B12 deficiency
- Folate deficiency

Vitamin B12 deficiency:

- Impaired vitamin B12 absorption in gut:
  - o Pancreatic insufficiency
  - o Blindloop syndrome
  - o Surgical resection
- Dietary deficiency:
  - o Pernicious anemia
  - o Gastrectomy
  - o Strict vegetarian

Folic acid deficiency:

- Increased requirement:
  - o Pregnancy
  - o Chronic hemolytic anemia
- Dietary deficiency:
  - o Drugs
  - o Tropical sprue
  - o Decreased absorption

Laboratory features:

- Hypersegmented neutrophils
- Increased LDH
- Giant platelets

Management:

- Associated neurological condition: SACD of spinal cord
- It is advised to give vitamin B12 and folic acid concurrently because treatment with folate alone may improve anemia but leads to progression of neurological disease

SICKLE CELL ANEMIA

Pathology:

- Replacement of glutamate by valine at 6 beta chain of HbA (point mutation)
- Autosomal recessive
- HbS heterozygotes are protected from malaria (falciparum)
- Thrombotic crisis/painful crisis/vaso-occlusive crisis is precipitated by:
  - o Infection,
  - o Dehydration
  - o Deoxygenation

- o Acidosis
- o Leads to polymerization of HbS, sickling of RBCs and hemolysis

Features:

- Asymptomatic
- Sickle cell crisis:
  - o Priapism
  - o Bone pain
  - o Chest pain
- Features of hemolysis:
  - o Pallor
  - o Jaundice
  - o Splenomegaly in early period

Lab findings:

- Features of hemolysis
- PBF shows:
  - o Target cells
  - o Sickle cells
- X-ray:
  - o Cod-fish mouth vertebrae/H-shaped vertebrae
  - o AVN/bone infarction
  - o Periosteal reaction (bone within bone appearance)

Complications:

- Salmonella osteomyelitis
- Aplastic crisis (parvovirus B19)
- Autosplenectomy
- Renal papillary necrosis (FSGN)
- Normocytic normochromic anemia

HEREDITARY SPHEROCYTOSIS

Basic pathology:

- Defect in ankyrin (50%); binds protein 3 and spectrin
- Genetic defect in RBC membrane
- RBC assumes a spherical shape and hemolysed (extravascular hemolysis)
- Inherited as: Autosomal dominant

Clinical features:

- Massive splenomegaly
- Anemia
- Jaundice
- Gallstones

Laboratory features:

- Low MCV
- Raised MCHC and osmotic fragility

Assessed by:

- Raised osmotic fragility of the RBC

Management:

- Splenectomy
- Howell Jolly bodies are seen after spleen removal

HEMOPHILIA

Features:

- Factor VIIIc deficiency/F8 gene mutation: Hemophilia A
- Factor IX deficiency/F9 gene mutation: Hemophilia B/ Christmas disease
- X-linked recessive (so patient is always a male)
- Recurrent bleeding into joints (hemarthroses) and muscles

Management:

- Replacement of deficient factors
- Antifibrinolytic agents (EACA, tranexamic acid)

HODGKIN'S LYMPHOMA

Features:

- Bimodal distribution (20's and 50's)
- Cervical lymphadenopathy (localized, single group)
- Centrifugal spread
- Constitutional features (B symptoms): Pel- Ebstein fever, night sweats, loss of weight
- Patients usually present in stage IIA
- Ann Arbor staging (prognostic)
- Less extranodal spread
- Causative agent: EBV
- Malignant cell is: Reed-Sternberg cell (B-cell origin, owl eye appearance)
- RS cell are positive for: CD 15, CD 30, except Lymphocytic predominant

Nodular sclerosis:

- Most common type
- Lacunar cells
- Collagen banding
- Affects females (Most common type in females)
- Very good prognosis

Mixed cellularity type:

- Most common type in India
- Numerous RS cells
- Good prognosis

Lymphocytic predominant:

- Best prognosis
- Popcorn cells (polypoidal)
- Histogenitically different subtype
- Lymphocytic predominant (negative for CD15, CD30) which is Positive for:
  - o CD20
  - o CD45

Regimes used (stage IIB-IV):

- ABVD:
  - o Adriamycin
  - o Bleomycin
  - o Vincristine
  - o Dacarbazine
- MOPP:
  - o Mechlorethamine
  - o Vincristine
  - o Procarbazine
  - o Prednisone

V. DISEASES OF THE GASTROINTESTINAL TRACT

H. PYLORI

Diseases caused:

- Gastritis
- Gastric Ca
- Peptic ulcer disease
- Gastric lymphoma

Test for documenting eradication:

- C^{13}/C^{14} Urea breath test:
  - o Non-invasive
  - o Simple
  - o Useful for follow-up

Test for epidemiology:

- Serology (not used for follow-up)

Tests for H. pylori:

- Non-invasive:
  - o Urea breath test
  - o Serology
  - o Stool antigen test
- Invasive:
  - o Rapid urease
  - o Culture
  - o Histology

Treatment of H. pylori:

- Quadruple therapy
- **TOMB**:
  - o Tetracycline
  - o Omeprazole
  - o Metronidazole
  - o Bismuth subsalicylate

Ulcers:

- Most common site of peptic ulcer: 1st part of duodenum
- Most common complication of peptic ulcer: Hemorrhage
- Most common site of Cushing's ulcer (seen in raised intracranial pressure): Stomach
- Curlings ulcer: Stress ulcer after burns

DUODENAL ULCER

Features:

- Blood group O
- Caused by H. pylori
- More common than gastric ulcer

- Pain 2-4 hours after eating/night pain/empty stomach
- Pain relieved by eating
- Normal gastrin levels
- Most common in: 1st portion of duodenum

WHIPPLE'S DISEASE

Features:

- Common in older men
- Arthralgia, neurologic and cardiac symptoms
- Specific test: Biopsy (PAS positive foamy macrophages in lamina propria of intestine)
- Caused by: Tropheryma whipplei
- Management by Cotrimoxazole/ceftriaxone

COELIAC DISEASE/GLUTEN SENSITIVE ENTEROPATHY

Features:

- HLA-DQ2
- Manifest within 1st year/3rd decade
- Sensitivity to protein gluten:
  - o Wheat
  - o Barley
  - o Rye
- Associated with dermatitis herpetiformis
- Antibodies:
  - o IgA antiendomysial
  - o Anti-tissue transglutaminase/tTGA (for screening)
  - o Anti-gliadin
- Diagnosed by:
  - o Immunology
  - o Jejunal biopsy
- Findings on jejunal biopsy:
  - o Total Villous atrophy (duodenal and jejunal villi)
  - o Crypt hyperplasia BUT thickness of mucosa unaltered
- Gluten free diet is recommended

ULCERATIVE COLITIS

Features:

- Toxic megacolon
- Pseudopolyps
- Involvement of bowel continuous from rectum
- Mucosal disease
- Affects colon only
- Usually bloody stool
- Crampy lower abdominal pain

Radiography:

- Loss of haustrations
- Shortening of bowel

Barium enema:

- Loss of haustrations (pipe stem colon)
- Pseudopolyps
- Shortening of bowel

CROHN'S DISEASE

Features:

- Skip lesions
- Creeping fat
- Antisachromyces cerevicase antibody/ASCA
- Usually discontinuous involvement of bowel (skip areas)
- Transmural disease
- Granulomas are sometimes seen
- May affects small and large bowel
- Mass felt in right lower quadrant
- Constant pain

Radiography:

- Narrowing of bowel lumen

Barium enema:

- Skip lesions
- Rose thorn appearance
- String sign
- Cobblestone

VI. DISEASES OF THE EXCRETORY SYSTEM

DIABETIC NEPHROPATHY

Features:

- Microalbuminuria: 30-299 mg/d (a risk factor for CVS disease)
- Macroalbuminuria: >300 mg/d
- After macroalbuminuria, GFR starts falling and end stage renal disease sets in 8-10 years

Histology:

- Most characteristic finding: Nodular glomerulosclerosis
- Most common finding: Diffuse glomerulosclerosis

Types:

- Type 1/IDDM
- IDDM presentation: Usually <25 years
- Ketoacidosis commoner in: IDDM
- Type 2/NIDDM
- HLA link of NIDDM: No links

Terms:

- Dawn phenomenon: Glucose level rise in early morning
- Somogyi effect: Rebound hyperglycemia may appear after 1-24 hours after moderate to severe hypoglycemia

Other points:

- Absence of chest pain in DM patients is: Silent ischemia (due to neuropathy)
- Parameter used to monitor long term DM control: HbA1c
- Parameter used to monitor short term DM control: Serum fructosamine
- Early test for DM nephropathy: Persistent micro-albuminuria (30-299 mg/d) in a 24 hour collection
- Kimmelstiel Wilson nodule: Characteristic histological feature of DM nephropathy

NEPHROTIC SYNDROME

Features:

- >3 gm/day proteinuria
- Hypoalbuminemia
- Edema
- Hypercoagulable states
- Hyperlipidemia and lipiduria

MINIMAL CHANGE DISEASE

Features:

- Seen in children <15 years
- 75% cases of nephrotic syndrome in children is because of MCD
- Selective proteinuria (LMW protein like albumin is excreted)
- Normal light microscopy
- Fusion of foot process on electron microscopy
- Remission of proteinuria with steroid therapy indicates a good prognosis
- Responds well to Steroids
- No deposits of complement/Ig (therefore also known as Nil deposit disease)
- Electron microscopy findings: Fusion/effacement/loss of foot process
- Changes on light microscopy: No change

VII. DISEASES OF THE ENDOCRINE SYSTEM

HYPOTHYROIDISM/HT

Types:

- Primary HT: Defect in thyroid gland
- Secondary HT: Pituitary gland is at fault

Primary hypothyroidism:

- Parameter:
  - o T3: Low
  - o T4: Low
  - o TSH: High
- Causes:
  - o Endemic goiter
  - o Amiodarone therapy

- o Goitrogens (cabbage)

Secondary hypothyroidism:

- Parameters:
  - o T3: Low
  - o T4: Low
  - o TSH: Low
- Causes:
  - o Sheehan syndrome (postpartum anterior pituitary necrosis)
  - o Empty sella syndrome

Clinical features (ABCDE):

- Alopecia
- Bradycardia
- Body temperature is less (subnormal)
- Cold intolerance
- Constipation
- Cool peripheral extremities
- Carpal tunnel syndrome
- Cavity (serous) effusions
- Dry skin
- Difficulty in concentration
- Dyspnea
- Delayed relaxation of deep tendon reflexes (hung-up reflexes)
- Edema (peripheral)
- Edema (myxedema)

PRIMARY HYPERPARATHYROIDISM

Most common cause:

- Solitary adenoma (80%)

Features:

- Bones (brown tumour)
- Stones (renal calculi)
- Abdominal groans (peptic ulcer)
- Psychic moans (depression)

Blood chemistry:

- Raised Ca
- Low phosphate
- Normal/increased alkaline phosphatase

CONN'S SYNDROME

Basic pathology:

- Hyperaldosteronism

Features:

- Due to adrenal adenoma or Ca
- No pedal edema
- Expansion of plasma volume
- Hypertension (diastolic)
- Decreased K^+ (muscle cramps and fatigue)
- Polyuria, polydypsia
- Proximal myopathy

Investigations:

- Increased sodium
- Decreased potassium

ECG:

- Prominent U waves (due to hypokalemia)

IOC:

- Plasma renin/aldosterone ratio

Treatment:

- Surgical removal of tumour
- Spironolactone

ADDISON'S DISEASE

Pathology:

- Primary adrenocortical insufficiency

Etiopathology:

- Decrease in aldosterone, corticosteroids and sex steroids
- Causes:
  - o TB (Most common cause in India)
  - o Autoimmune (Most common cause worldwide)
  - o Addisonian crisis (sudden stoppage of steroid drugs)
  - o Waterhouse-Friderichsen syndrome
  - o Sheehan syndrome
- Drug associated with Addisonian like features: Busulfan

Clinical features:

- Low:
  - o Sugar (hypoglycemia)

- o Salt (salt wasting because of loss of water and salt)
- o Mean BP
- High:
  - o Urine output (polyuria >3L/day)
  - o Potassium (hyperkalemia and metabolic acidosis)
  - o ACTH (hyperpigmentation)

Metabolic effects:

- Hyperkalemia
- Hyponatremia
- Increased pigmentation (increase in ACTH, which behaves like melanocyte stimulating hormone) (EXCEPT in secondary adrenal insufficiency due to pituitary failure)

Investigation:

- Low sodium
- High potassium

ECG:

- Tall peaked/tented T waves (because of hyperkalemia)

Definitive investigation:

- ACTH stimulation test/cosyntropin test

Management:

- To promote salt and water retention: Fludrocortisone
- To reduce hypoglycemic symptoms: Dexamethasone
- For Addison disease: Hydrocortisone
- For Addisonian crisis: Fluid resuscitation and hydrocortisone

VIII. DISEASES OF THE NERVOUS SYSTEM

Alzheimer's disease:

- Most common cause of dementia in elderly: Alzheimer's disease
- Presenile dementia occurs before the age of: 60 years
- Useful screening test for dementia: Mini mental status examination
- Maximum score in mini mental status examination: 30

GUILLAIN-BARRÉ SYNDROME

Feature:

- Ascending type of motor paralysis
- Arreflexia
- Flaccidity

CSF examination:

- Albuminocytological dissociation (increase in protein without an increase in cells)

Treatment:

- Plasmapheresis
- Immunoglobulin

CEREBELLAR LESION

Features:

- Ataxia/asynergia (inability to do movements smoothly and accurately)
- Intention tremor (NOT resting ones)
- Head tremors/head tilt/intentional tremors
- Pendular knee jerk/decreased deep tendon reflexes
- Hypotonia
- Nystagmus
- Dysarthria (staccato speech)
- Ataxia with leaning towards side of lesion
- Dysdiadochokinesia (rapid alternating movements)
- Dysmetria/past pointing

MENINGITIS

Most common cause:

- Neonatal meningitis:
  - o Gram negative bacilli (E. coli): India
  - o Group B Streptococcus: Worldwide
- Most common cause of meningitis in adults: S. pneumonia

Bacterial meningitis:

- CSF findings:
  - o Purulent exudates
  - o Cloudy CSF

- o Decreased glucose (<2.2 mmol/L)
- o Increased protein concentration (>0.45 g/L)
- Cells: Neutrophils (>1000 cells)

Viral meningitis:

- Most commonly caused by: Enterovirus (80-90%)
- CSF findings:
  - o Lymphocytic pleocytosis (>25/cubic mm)
  - o Normal glucose level
  - o Normal/mildly elevated CSF pressure

INFECTIONS

Neurosyphilis:

- Tract involved: Dorsal column
- Features:
  - o Sensory loss
  - o Argyll Robertson pupil
  - o Bladder dysfunction
- Associated term: Tabes dorsalis

OTHER CONDITIONS AFFECTING NERVOUS SYSTEM

Neuropathic joint disease:

- Most common cause of neuropathic joint disease: DM
- Most common joint affected by DM: Tarsal joints
- Other associated conditions:
  - o Leprosy
  - o Syringomyelia
  - o Tabes dorsalis

PARKINSONISM

Features:

- 2nd most common neurodegenerative disease
- Intracytoplasmic proteinaceous inclusions known as Lewy bodies
- Parkinson disease is the most common form of parkinsonism

Pathology:

- Symptoms of parkinsonism are due to: Loss of nerve cells in substantia nigra pars compacta (SNc) and the locus coeruleus (midbrain)
- Drugs causing parkinsonism:
  - o Methyl dopa
  - o Reserpine
  - o Metoclopramide

Features:

- Cardinal features:
  - o Resting tremor
    - – Most common manifestation
    - – Occurs at rest
    - – Worsens with emotional stress
  - o Bradykinesia
  - o Rigidity, gait disturbance/postural instability (Festinating gait)
- Other features:
  - o Masked facies
  - o Reduced eye blink
  - o Dysphagia

Treatment:

- Levodopa + peripheral decarboxylase inhibitor
- MAO (monoamine oxidase)-B inhibitors: Selegiline

SUBARACHNOID HEMORRHAGE

Clinical presentation:

- 60 years old patient with severe headache and neck stiffness of abrupt onset
- She had never such a severe headache before
- She may have photophobia and nausea

Subarachnoid hemorrhage CSF findings:

- Pressure and proteins: Increased
- Colour: Red stained
- Cells: RBC
- Sugar: Normal

IX. CONNECTIVE TISSUE DISORDERS

SLE

Pathology:

- Multisystem autoimmune disorder
- Normocytic normochromic anemia
- LE cells

Features:

- Butterfly rash/malar rash (photosensitivity)
- False positive test for syphilis
- Libman-Sacks endocarditis
- Musculoskeletal finding: Non-erosive arthritis
- Renal manifestations: Wire loop lesions (diffuse proliferative lupus nephritis)
- Pulmonary system findings: Shrinking lung syndrome
- Most common cause of death: Renal involvement

Specific antibody for SLE:

- Anti-ds DNA (very specific and denotes poor prognosis)
- Anti-Sm antibodies are also highly specific but lack sensitivity
- ANA is 95% sensitive but not specific
- Anti-histone antibodies in drug induced lupus (**HIP**: Hydralazine, INH, procainamide)

X. DISORDERS AFFECTING MUSCLES

DUCHENNE MUSCULAR DYSTROPHY

Pathology:

- Inheritance: X linked recessive
- Defect lies in which gene: Dystrophin gene
- Pathology in which protein: Sarcolemmal protein defect

Features:

- Pseudohypertrophy of muscles
- Gowers sign: Patient, while standing, tries to climb on himself

MYASTHENIA GRAVIS/MG

Pathology:

- Autoimmune
- Bimodal (30-40 is women; 70-80s in men)
- Decreased myoneural junction transmission (anti-Acetylcholine receptor antibodies)

Types:

- Generalised MG:
  - o Bulbar
  - o Facial
- Ocular MG:
  - o Ptosis
  - o Diplopia

Investigation:

- Edrophonium/Tensilon test (acetylcholinesterase inhibitor)
- Single fiber EMG: Most sensitive

Features:

- Dysarthria
- Dysphagia
- Fatiguable chewing (bulbar)
- Proximal muscle weakness (muscle weakness and fatigability which worsens by the end of the day)
- Normal: Sensory modalities and deep tendon reflexes

Treatment:

- Most commonly used cholinergic drugs: Pyridostigmine/Neostigmine (acetylcholinesterase inhibitor)
- Surgical procedure (should be done in all cases): Thymectomy

XI. HEPATOLOGY

HEPATITIS

Hepatitis:

- Spreading by feco-oral route:
  - o HAV
  - o HEV
- Most common cause of sporadic hepatitis in adults: HEV
- Worst prognosis in pregnancy: HEV
- Most prone to chronicity: HCV

Markers of HBV:

- First viral marker to appear after HBV infection: HBsAg
- Indicator of intrahepatic viral replication/presence of which marker indicates high infectivity:
  - o HBeAg
  - o HBV DNA
- Recent infection of HBV is indicated by: IgM anti-HBcAg
- HBsAg appears first (declines by 3-6 months)
- HBeAg, HBV-DNA and DNA polymerase are markers of active viral replication
- Persistence of HBeAg: Continued viral replication and infectivity and progression to chronicity
- IgM anti-HBc: First antibody to appear followed by anti-Hbe
- Anti-HBe: Suggests recovery (good prognosis)
- IgG anti-HBc: Slowly replaces the IgM over months

WILSON DISEASE

Pathology:

- AR inheritance
- Genetic defect on chromosome 13
- Neuropsychiatric disorder
- Sunflower cataract

Features:

- Hepatic dysfunction
- Eye changes (KF rings in descemet's membrane of cornea) and
- Neurologic manifestations (NO sensory changes)

Investigations:

- Serum ceruloplasmin: Low
- Total serum copper: Low
- Free copper: High
- Urine copper excretion: >1.6 mmol/day
- Liver biopsy: Copper concentration >250 microgram/gm of dry tissue
- KF rings: Present in all patients

Treatment:

- Drug used as alternative to zinc: Trientine (2nd DOC)
- Drug for maintenance therapy: Zinc acetate/gluconate (1st DOC)

SECTION 5: SURGICAL DISORDERS

I. ARTERIAL AND VENOUS DISORDERS

THROMBOANGITIS OBLITERANS/ BUERGER'S DISEASE

Buerger's disease:

- It is a vaso-occlusive disease of the small and medium size arteries and veins commonly affecting the lower limb of young male smoker
- Smoking is a strong contributory factor
- Medium and small size vessels (arteries and veins) are affected
- Segmental involvement of vessels

Clinical features:

- Male smoker 20-30 years of age
- Most common in lower limbs
- Migrating thrombophlebitis
- First symptom: Numbness and coldness in feet/toes

Other features of arterial occlusion:

- Intermittent claudication
- Rest pain
- Colour changes
- Ulceration
- Gangrene

Investigations:

- Doppler USG
- Low ankle pressure index is low (ankle SBP/arm SBP; normally >1)

Arteriography:

- Multiple occluded segments in small and medium sized arteries
- Corkscrew appearance because of development of collateral circulation
- Martorell's sign (fine, tortuous vessels, replacing the diseased arteries due to opening of collaterals)
- Fine collaterals are displayed as tree root or spider leg appearance on arteriography

Management:

- Stop smoking
- Relief of pain: Vasodilators (phentolamine/phenoxy-benzamine), pentoxyfylline, xanthinol nicotinate, analgesic, paravertebral or common peroneal nerve block

Lumbar sympathectomy done if:

- Rest pain
- Ischemic ulceration not responding to conservative treatment
- Preserve L1 (otherwise dry ejaculation may occur)

Amputation:

- If the lumbar sympathectomy fail to heal the ulcers and gangrenous lesions of the limb
- Omentopexy
- Arteriovenous/AV fistula (between popliteal artery and popliteal vein)

DEEP VENOUS THROMBOSIS

DVT:

- Venous thrombi is mainly composed of RBC and fibrin whereas arterial thrombi are mainly formed of platelets

Virchow's triad:

- Stasis of blood
- Trousseau's sign (hypercoagulability of blood)
- Changes in endothelial lining of vessel wall

Phlegmasia

- Phlegmasia alba dolens/white leg: Deep femoral vein thrombosis associated with lymphangitis

- Phlegmasia caerulea dolens/blue leg: Extensive DVT of iliac and pelvic veins

Features:

- Most common site: Calf veins
- Earliest sign of DVT: Rise in temperature
- Clinical presentation:
  - o Unilateral leg swelling
  - o Local warmth
  - o Erythema
  - o Pain
- Homan's sign in DVT: Forced dorsiflexion of foot causes calf pain

Investigations:

- Contrast phlebography (gold standard)
- Fibrinogen uptake test
- Duplex USG:
  - o Investigation of choice
  - o Allows accurate visualization of deep vein
  - o Makes a positive diagnosis of DVT

Management:

- Bed rest
- Anticoagulation (Heparin/warfarin)
  - o LMW Heparin: Decreased dosing schedule and less risk of heparin induced thrombocytopenia
- Aspirin
- Calf length pneumatic compression devices
- Thrombolytic therapy (streptokinase/urokinase)
- Operative thrombectomy

VARICOSE VEINS

2 types:

- Primary varicose veins: Incompetent valve in superficial system alone; may be inherited
- Secondary varicose veins: Incompetent communicating and deep veins of the leg

Features:

- Varicose veins are dilated, tortuous superficial veins
- Most common site is leg
- Test to demonstrate saphenofemoral incompetence
  - o Brodie-Trendelenburg (I) test
  - o Trendelenberg II for perforator incompetence

Gold standard investigation:

- Duplex imaging

Management:

- Palliative: Elastic stockings/bandage
- Sclerosant injection: 5% Ethanolamine oleate (injection given to promote thrombosis and sclerosis of veins)
- Surgery:
  - o Saphenofemoral flush ligation: For long saphenous varicosity
  - o Popliteal flush ligation: For short saphenous varicosity
- Cockett and Dodd operation: For incompetent communicating veins

II. WOUND AND TISSUE REPAIR

Healing by primary/1st intention:

- Closed wounds
- Edges approximated
- Example: Clean skin incision closed with sutures
- Clean cut wound with edges approximated, no infection

Healing by secondary intention:

- Wound is infected, edges not approximated properly and significant tissue loss is present
- Slow healing
- More scar formation

Factors delaying wound healing:

- Vitamin C deficiency
- Deficiency of trace metals (zinc, copper etc.)
- Absence of oxygen (reduced perfusion)
- Presence of vitamin E (inhibitory role)
- Anemia
- Infection etc.

Sutures:

- Absorbable sutures:
  - o Catgut
  - o Dexon (polyglycolic acid)
- Non absorbable sutures:
  - o Prolene
  - o Silk

SKIN GRAFTS

Partial thickness (Thiersch) grafts:

- Contains epidermis + upper capillary dermis
- Vascularized by ingrowth of capillaries from underlying tissue

Full thickness (Wolfe) graft:

- Contains epidermis + whole of dermis
- Has normal skin texture and reduced tendency of contracture
- 'Take' is also reduced
- Can be taken from areas of thin skin (ear, upper eyelid or scalp)

Composite grafts:

- Consist of skin and some underlying tissue (fat, cartilage etc.)

III. SALIVARY GLANDS

Pleomorphic adenoma:

- Most common tumor of parotid
- Mixed parotid tumor (Cartilage + epithelial cells)
- Most common in females
- Usually present as solitary mass
- Firm, lobulated, painless swelling over parotid region
- Free from skin and deeper tissues (masseter)
- No involvement of facial nerve
- Superficial lobe is usually involved
- Most common malignancy developing in pleomorphic adenoma is adenocarcinoma (otherwise in a normal parotid, it is mucoepidermoid Ca)
- Malignant transformation (seen in 2-10%) is suggested if:
  - o Feels stony hard
  - o Facial nerve is involved
  - o Fixed to skin or deeper tissue
  - o Swelling grows rapidly
  - o Becomes painful
  - o Involvement of cervical lymph nodes
- Diagnosis is made by needle biopsy (per oral route)
- Most common benign parotid gland tumour: Pleomorphic adenoma (Most common benign tumour of major and minor salivary glands)
- Treatment of pleomorphic adenoma: Superficial parotidectomy (Patey's operation)
- Surgical procedure done is superficial/partial parotidectomy with conservation of facial nerve

For better preparation and success in AIIMS-NORCET Exam, download **'drkamalkvgroup'** mobile app from Google Playstore.

WhatsApp: +91 84 7000 4333

IV. BREAST

CARCINOMA BREAST

Aetiology:

- More common in developed Western worls
- Risk factors for breast Ca:
  - o Positive family history
  - o Nullipara
  - o Attaining early menarche and late menopause have high-risk
  - o Early child-bearing and breastfeeding reduces the risk
  - o Obese
  - o Benign breast disease with atypia, hyperplasia and epitheliosis has got higher risk
  - o Most common in individuals who are on oral contraceptive pills and hormone replacement therapy for more than 5 years
- BRCA:
  - o BRCA 1: 17q (long arm of chromosome 17)
  - o BRCA 2: 13q (long arm of chromosome 13)

Features:

- Most common site: Upper outer quadrant
- Peau'd orange:
  - o Due to obstruction of dermal lymphatics, opening of the sebaceous glands and hair follicles get buried in the oedema giving rise to orange peel appearance
- Nipple retraction
- Dimpling of skin due to infiltration of ligament of Cooper
- Ulceration and discharge from nipple and areola

Investigations:

- Breast Imaging Reporting and Data System for mammographic findings (BIRADS grading)
- Triple examination (PCR):
  - o **P**athological examination
  - o **C**linical examination
  - o **R**adiological examination
- MRI:
  - o Screening of breast carcinoma in high risk cases
- Mammography:
  - o Used for screening in old age
  - o Carries risk of radiation so not used in reproductive age group
- Best prognostic factor is status of lymph nodes

Management:

- Treatment of Estrogen receptor positive (ER+) in a premenopausal women: Tamoxifen (Tamoxifen increases risk of uterine Ca)
- Management of stage I and II of breast Ca: Lumpectomy/breast conservative therapy + axillary clearance + radiotherapy

V. HEAD AND NECK

THYROGLOSSAL CYST

Most common site:

- Beneath the hyoid
- Occupies the midline usually (except in the region of thyroid cartilage)

Feature:

- Swelling moves upwards on protrusion of the tongue
- Also moves on swallowing (attachment with foramen caecum)

For better preparation and success in AIIMS-NORCET Exam, download **'drkamalkvgroup'** mobile app from Google Playstore.

WhatsApp: +91 84 7000 4333

VI. THYROID

MEN SYNDROME

MEN-I/Wermer syndrome:

- Parathyroid neoplasm
- Pancreas neoplasm
- Pituitary (anterior) adenoma

MEN-IIA/Sipple syndrome:

- Medullary Ca (thyroid)
- Phaeochromocytomas
- Parathyroid hyperplasia

MEN-IIB:

- Medullary Ca (thyroid)
- Phaeochromocytomas
- Mucosal neuromas (with distinctive Marfanoid habitus)
- Parathyroid (rare)

THYROID TUMOURS

Medullary Ca:

- Occurrence: 80% cases are sporadic
- Mode of inheritance: 20% are familial (MEN-IIa or MEN-IIb)
- Histological feature: Stroma of MTC shows material with staining properties of amyloid
- Characteristic histological feature: MTC can be diagnosed by demonstrating calcitonin within the MTC cells (on immunohistochemical studies)
- Management: Total thyroidectomy is the TOC

Papillary Ca:

- Most common thyroid tumour
- Encapsulated

- Psammoma bodies are seen
- Multifocal
- Least malignant

Thyroidectomy:

- Neck swelling immediately following thyroid surgery is due to: Tension hematoma (so open immediately)

VII. DISEASES OF THE GASTROINTESTINAL TRACT

MALLORY-WEISS SYNDROME

Common in:

- Alcoholics

Most common site:

- Cardia of stomach (NOT esophagus)

Pathology:

- Partial vertical tears
- Pylorus closed and closed lower esophageal sphincter/LES (barotrauma)

Feature:

- Hematemesis

BOERHAAVE'S SYNDROME

Mechanism:

- Forceful vomiting (against a closed glottis)
- May produce perforation of the esophagus (transverse, posterolateral part)
- Cricopharynx and pylorus are closed

Clinical presentation:

- Presents with acute chest pain

ACHALASIA CARDIA

Clinical feature:

- Dysphagia is the presenting symptom
- Initially for liquids but later on for both liquids and solids

Pathology:

- Failure of relaxation of lower esophageal sphincter/LES

Manometric findings:

- Increased pressure in LES

Barium study shows:

- Bird beak appearance

IHPS/IDIOPATHIC HYPERTROPHIC PYLORIC STENOSIS

Presents at:

- About 4 weeks after birth
- Never congenital, therefore terminology has been changed from congenital HPS to idiopathic HPS

Feature:

- Weight loss
- Projectile vomiting
- Hypochloremic hypokalemic metabolic alkalosis

Fluid of choice:

- Isotonic Dextrose normal saline

GASTRIC CA

Most common site:

- Pylorus and Antrum

Predisposing factors:

- Organism: H. Pylori (causes gastritis, gastric atrophy)
- Blood group: A blood group
- Long term nitrates ingestion (dried, smoked, salted foods)
- Pernicious anemia
- Meneterier's disease
- Atrophic gastritis

Most common feature:

- Weight loss
- Virchow nodes/Troissier's sign
- Krunkenberg tumour
- Sister Mary Joseph node
- Blummer shelf (Pouch of Douglas)
- Linitis plastica

Early gastric Ca:

- Primary lesion limited to mucosa and submucosa
- Excellent prognosis

Sister Mary Joseph nodule:

- Metastatic involvement of paraumbilical nodes from intra-pelvic/intraabdominal malignancies (stomach)

DUODENAL ULCER

Pathology:

- Most common site of duodenal ulcer: Duodenal cap (anterior wall)
- Source of bleeding in duodenal ulcer: Gastroduodenal artery

Management of duodenal ulcer:

- Highly selective vagotomy/Proximal gastric vagotomy/ parietal cell vagotomy is done to reduce down chances of (complications) diarrhea/dumping syndrome
- Vagotomy and antrectomy is (Billroth I/II) done to lower down chances of recurrence

Treatment of perforated duodenal ulcer:

- NBM (Nil by mouth)
- Exploratory laparotomy
- Nasogastric suction
- Acid suppression
- Antibiotics

APPENDIX

Appendicitis:

- Pelvic and post-ileal appendicitis presents as: Diarrhea
- Most tender area: McBurney's point
- Imaging modalities: CECT confirmatory (but diagnosis is clinical)
- Managed by appendicectomy

Appendicular carcinoid:

- Most common malignant tumour of appendix
- Most common in distal third of appendix
- <1 cm
- Rarely metastasize
- Management: Appendicectomy

MECKEL'S DIVERTICULUM

Feature:

- True congenital diverticulum
- Vestigeal remnant of omphalomesenteric duct/vitelline duct
- 2 feet from ileocaecal valve
- 2 types of ectopic tissue are common (Gastric and pancreatic)

Complication:

- Torsion may lead to obstruction, ischemia and necrosis
- It can be a leading point of intussusception

IOC:

- Technetium-99m pertechnetate (99mTc)

INTUSSUSCEPTION

Features:

- Outer tube is known as: Intussuscipiens
- Inner tube is known as: Intussusceptum
- Sign de dance: Emptiness in Iliac fossa
- Most common type: Ileo-colic

COLORECTAL CA

Pathology:

- Most common site: Rectum
- Most common site in colon: Sigmoid colon
- Most common type (histology): AdenoCa

Presentation:

- Right sided tumour: Anemia
- Left sided tumour presents as: Obstruction/pain
- Most common site of metastasis: Liver (33% patient may have metastasis)

Risk factors:

- Increased dietary fats and oil
- Elevated serum cholesterol
- Ulcerative colitis and Crohn's disease
- Familial adenomatous polyps

Treatment of choice:

- Surgery

VIII. HERNIA

Types:

- Spigelian hernia: Interparietal hernia (sub-umbilical/level of arcuate line)
- Littres hernia: Hernia of Meckel's diverticulum
- Morgagni's hernia: Hernia between costal and sternal parts of diaphragm

HERNIA EN GLISSADE/SLIDING HERNIA

Content on:

- Left side are: Sigmoid colon and mesentry
- Right side are: Caecum

FEMORAL HERNIA

Features:

- Most common in Female
- Most common on Right side
- Most common strangulates

IX. PANCREAS

ACUTE PANCREATITIS

Causes:

- Gallstones
- Alcoholism
- Investigation which can cause acute pancreatitis: ERCP

Abdominal signs:

- Cullen sign and Grey turner sign: Blue-red-purple or green-brown discoloration due to catabolism of hemoglobin

Diagnostic modality:

- CT scan

Prognosis:

- Best prognosis: Gallstone pancreatitis
- Recurrent pancreatitis occurs in: Methyl malonic acidemia

Conditions with raised serum amylase:

- Pancreatitis
- Ruptured ectopic pregnancy
- Parotitis
- Biliary peritonitis (duodenal injuries)
- Mesenteric infarction

PANCREATIC CA

Pathology:

- Most consistent risk factor: Cigarette smoking
- Most common site: Pancreatic head (70%)

Most common symptom:

- Weight loss and pain

INSULINOMA

Feature:

- Most common endocrine tumours of pancreas (from beta cells)
- Usually single
- Whipple's triad is seen
- Distributed equally throughout pancreas
- Total capsule removal is ensured to prevent tumour recurrence

For better preparation and success in AIIMS-NORCET Exam, download **'drkamalkvgroup'** mobile app from Google Playstore.

WhatsApp: +91 84 7000 4333

X. SPLEEN

SPLENECTOMY

Indications:

- Hereditary spherocytosis
- Portal hypertension

- Hypersplenism
- Sickle cell anemia

Splenectomy increases risk for:

- Pneumococcal infections
- H. Influenzae infections

Overwhelming post-splenectomy infection/OPSI:

- Most commonly caused by: Streptococcus pneumonia
- Most common complication: Left lower lobe atelectasis

XI. LIVER

Anatomy:

- Couinoud's segments are based on: Based on hepatic vein and portal vein division
- Segment I is: Segment I is caudate lobe
- Segmemt IV is: Segment IV is quadrate lobe
- Vascular supply of segment I: Independent vascular supply

Portal vein:

- Formed behind neck of pancreas, by union of splenic vein and superior mesenteric vein
- Portal hypertension: More than 12 mm Hg
- Sites of portosystemic anastomosis:
  - o Rectum and anal canal (hemorrhoids)
  - o Lower end of esophagus (varices)

AMOEBIC LIVER ABSCESS

Most common site:

- Right lobe (posterosuperior surface)

Characteristic of pus:

- Anchovy sauce pus (chocolate coloured pus due to RBC lysis)

Complications:

- Pleuropulmonary involvement
- Rupture into pleural space

HYDATID DISEASE

ELISA:

- ELISA is sensitive

Blood culture:

- No role of blood culture

Naked eye appearance:

- Crumbled egg appearance/white of a hard boiled egg

Technique used for management:

- PAIR technique

Steps in PAIR technique:

- Percutaneous Aspiration
- Injection of scolicidal agent
- Reaspiration of cyst contents

Most effective drug:

- Albendazole

PYOGENIC LIVER ABSCESS

Features:

- Usually single and large

Most common route of infection:

- Infection through bile duct (hematogenous route is 2nd most common route)

HEPATOCELLULAR CARCINOMA

Predisposing factors:

- HBV, HCV
- Alcoholic liver disease

Most common marker for HCC:

- AFP

Other markers:

- Neurotensin
- PIVKA 2

Imaging modalities:

- Screening: USG
- Percutaneous biopsy (USG/CT guided) can be diagnostic

Fibrolamellar Ca:

- Not associated with cirrhosis
- Slow growing
- Good prognosis, if treated

Indications for liver transplantation:

- Children: Biliary atresia
- Adults:
  - o Primary sclerosing cholangitis
  - o Fulminant hepatitis etc.

XII. GALLBLADDER

CHOLELITHIASIS

Pigment stones:

- Chronic hemolysis
- Alcoholic cirrhosis
- Chronic biliary tract infection

Complications of gallstones:

- Acute and chronic cholecystitis
- Carcinoma of gallbladder
- Acute pancreatitis
- Gallstone ileus (acute intestinal obstruction)

CBD stones:

- Most common cause of obstructive jaundice: CBD stone
- On USG, finding suggestive of CBD stone: Bile duct diameter of more than 6 mm
- Sign seen on cholangiography: Meniscus sign

XIII. GENITOURINARY SYSTEM

RENAL CALCULI

Types and features:

- Most common stones: Calcium stones (75-85%)
- Radiolucent stones: Uric acid
- Stones most common in men: Calcium
- Stones most common in females: Struvite stones
- Stones most common in UTI with urease producing bacteria (proteus spp.): Struvite stones
- Stone which grows in alkaline urine: Struvite stones
- Stone which grow in infected urine: Struvite stone
- Stone hard to break in ESWL: Cystine stones
- Pain in ureteric calculi is due to: Ureteric peristalsis

X-ray:

- Location of renal stone on lateral view of lumbar spine: Renal calculi overlies spine in lateral view

Dietl's crisis:

- Renal colic
- Swelling in loin
- Disappearance of swelling with micturition

URINARY BLADDER CARCINOMA

Most common type:

- Transitional cell Ca

Pure squamous Ca may be seen in:

- Seen when squamous metaplasia or keratinisation has occurred Schistosomiasis (vesical bilharziasis)

Earliest and Most common symptom:

- Painless hematuria

Vaccine used in initial stages (trial):

- BCG (intravesical)

URETHRA

Most common cause of urethral stricture:

- Trauma

Part of urethra injured in pelvic fracture:

- Membranous urethra

Mechanism of urethral injury:

- Fall astride a projecting object (History of blow to perineum)

Triad of ruptured bulbar urethra:

- Retention of urine
- Perineal hematoma
- Bleeding from external urinary meatus

Precaution in such cases:

- Avoid catheterization

HYPOSPADIAS

Associated terms:

- Hooded prepuce
- Meatal stenosis
- Bifid scrotum

Best time of surgery:

- Stage I: Managing chordee (Straightening of penis) at 18-24 months of age
- Stage II: Reconstruction of urethra at 5-7 years

INCOMPLETE DESCENT OF ESTES

Complication:

- Malignant change (even if the testes have been brought down surgically)

Best time to operate:

- Orchidopexy at 1 year

VARICOCELE

Most common on:

- Left side

Transillumination test is:

- Negative

Feature:

- Most common cause of male infertility, which is surgically treated

PROSTATE GLAND

Pathology:

- Carcinoma arises from: Peripheral zone
- BPH arises from: Periurethral zone

TURP for BPH:

- Most common complication of TURP: Retrograde ejaculation
- Irrigation fluid used in TURP: 1.5% glycine
- Drowsiness and altered sensorium after TURP may point toward: Hyponatremia

CARCINOMA PROSTATE

McNeals zone:

- Ca zone

Earliest marker/screening test:

- PSA

Metastasis to vertebrae is via:

- Batesons vertebral venous plexus

Staging system:

- Gleasons staging

Most sensitive test for screening of prostate Ca:

- Digital rectal examination
- PSA

XIV. SKIN TUMOURS

BASAL CELL CARCINOMA/RODENT ULCER

Features:

- Arises from epidermal basal cells
- Locally invasive (no lymphatic/blood stream dissemination)
- Most common form of skin Ca
- Sunlight is predisposing factor
- Usual site is face, usually above a line joining the ear lobule to the angle of the mouth
- Most common site: Face/Inner canthus of eyes
- White races
- Unknown in black

Most common type of BCC:

- Noduloulcerative type

Mode of spread:

- Direct
- Very slow growing
- Most common low grade malignancy of Head and neck region

Excision procedure done:

- Moh's micrographic excision
- Highly radiosensitive
- Excision with healthy margin can be done

XV. MISCELLANOUS

TOTAL PARENTERAL NUTRITION

TPN is used as a primary therapy in:

- Indicated in patients with compromised gut functions who require nutritional therapy for > 10 days
- Severe burns
- Short bowel syndrome

Complications of TPN:

- Air embolism (most fatal)
- Weight loss in 7 days

Metabolic changes in TPN:

- Essential fatty acid deficiency
- Electrolyte disorder (hyperkalemic hyperchloremic metabolic acidosis) etc.

SECTION 6: BASICS OF ORTHOPEDICS

I. GENERAL ORTHOPEDICS

Fractures and eponyms:

- Greenstick fracture:
  - o Children
  - o Bending force
  - o Distraction of cortex on convex side and compression on the concave side (cortex intact)
- Bennet's fracture: Intra-articular base of 1st metacarpal
- Rolando's fracture: Intra-articular fracture base of first metacarpal with comminution
- Jefferson's fracture: Burst fracture of C1 (atlas)
- Hangman's fracture: Traumatic spondylolisthesis of cervical vertebrae 2
- Monteggia fracture: Proximal ulna fracture with dislocation of proximal superior radioulnar joint
- Galeazzi fracture: Galeazzi is fracture distal radius with dislocation of distal radioulnar joint
- March fracture: Stress fracture of shaft of 2nd or 3rd metatarsal (commonly)
- Pott's fracture: Bimalleolar fracture

Fracture healing:

- Most important factor for fracture healing: Degree of immobilization
- Stages in fracture healing:
  - o Hematoma
  - o Granulation tissue
  - o Callus formation
  - o Modelling
  - o Remodelling

Most common Fractures

- Most common fracture in childhood: Distal humeral fracture (Supracondylar fracture)
- Most common bone fracture in body: Clavicle
- Most common bone fracture during birth: Clavicle

Bursitis

- Infrapatellar bursitis: Clergyman's knee
- Prepatellar bursitis: Housemaid's knee
- Olecranon bursitis: Student's elbow

Casts and uses

- Tube/Cylindrical cast: Knee fracture
- Cast in glass holding position: Scaphoid fracture
- PTB cast: Tibial fracture

Splints

- Cock up splint: Radial nerve injury
- Aeroplane splint: Brachial plexus injury
- Von Rosen splint: CDH/DDH (Developmental dysplasia of hip)

II. INJURIES OF UPPER LIMB

DISLOCATION SHOULDER

Features:

- Shoulder joint is the most common joint to dislocate
- Shoulder joint is the most common joint to undergo recurrent dislocation
- Most common mechanism of injury is FOSH (fall on outstretched hand) with shoulder externally rotated
- Most common type: Subcoracoid type (Anterior dislocation)

Management:

- Managed by closed reduction by Kocher's manoeuvre
- Steps are TEAM (traction, external rotation, adduction and medial/internal rotation)

Complications:

- Axillary nerve damage
- Recurrent dislocation

COLLE'S FRACTURE

Features:

- Fracture occurs at the corticocancellous junction of the lower end of radius
- Usually seen in elderly post-menopausal women are at risk (because of osteoporosis)
- Normally radial styloid process is at a lower level than ulnar styloid process, but in Colle's fracture, radial styloid process comes to lie at the same level or at a higher level than ulnar styloid process
- Characteristic deformity: Dinner fork deformity
- Patient is managed by closed reduction and application of cast (in palmar flexion and ulnar deviation)
- Finger stiffness is the most common complication

SCAPHOID FRACTURE

Features:

- Only carpal bone to undergo fracture as well as AVN/ avascular necrosis: Scaphoid
- Fragment undergoing necrosis in fracture scaphoid: Proximal
- Most common site of fracture scaphoid: Waist
- Clinically patient comes with pain and tenderness over anatomical snuff box after a FOSH (**f**all **o**n **o**utstretched **h**and)
- Initial X-rays does not show fracture and hence diagnosis is always clinical
- Oblique views should be done at the time of injury and after 2 weeks to look for fracture line
- Managed by scaphoid cast application in glass holding position

VOLKMAN ISCHEMIA/COMPARTMENT SYNDROME

Compartment syndrome:

- Muscles are enclosed in an inelastic fascial compartment. If there is edema, it will compress muscles, which will lead to further edema and a vicious cycle continues
- This can be encountered in forearm and leg region particularly after injury and a tight cast application
- Most important sign of Volkmann ischemia/compartment syndrome: Passive stretch pain (when the fingers/toes are stretched dorsally)
- Management:
  - o If this is because of a tight cast, bivalve it or remove it
  - o In cases of impending compartment syndrome, one has to release the pressure on muscles by doing fasciotomy

III. INJURIES OF LOWER LIMB

Hip dislocation:

- Most common type: Posterior dislocation
- Attitude of limb in posterior dislocation is FADIR:
  - o **F**lexion
  - o **Ad**duction
  - o **I**nternal **R**otation
- Posterior hip dislocation commonly occurs because of dashboard injury (car)
- Emergency reduction needs to be done
- Can injure sciatic nerve

For better preparation and success in AIIMS-NORCET Exam, download **'drkamalkvgroup'** mobile app from Google Playstore.

WhatsApp: +91 84 7000 4333

IV. BONY TUMOURS

Location of tumours:

- Epiphyseal:
  - o Osteoclastoma
  - o Chondroblastoma
- Metaphyseal:
  - o Osteosarcoma
  - o Osteochondroma
  - o Aneurysmal bone cyst

- Diaphysis:
  - o Ewing's sarcoma
  - o Osteoid osteoma

V. INFECTIONS OF BONE

OSTEOMYELITIS

Acute Osteomyelitis/OM:

- Earliest site of involvement in primary OM: Metaphysis
  - o Because metaphysis is the growing highly vascular region of bone with hair-pin arrangement of vessels
- Diagnosis of acute OM: Blood culture (positive in 65% cases)
- Most common organism in acute OM: Staphylococcus aureus (In sickle cell anemia patients, OM is usually caused by salmonella)
- Most common site of acute OM in children: Lower femoral epiphysis
- Most common type of osteomyelitis: Secondary (from contiguous focus of infection because of open/compound fractures or bony operative procedures which get infected)
- In children, most common type is primary, which is hematogenous in origin
- Diagnosis of acute OM is always clinical
- Management is with broad spectrum antibiotics if the patient reports within 48 hours. Otherwise it is presumed that pus has formed and surgical exploration and drainage is needed

Chronic osteomyelitis:

- Chronic OM is the most common complication of untreated/inadequately treated OM
- Most common site is lower end of femur
- Most common presenting symptom is chronic discharging sinus
- Discharge of bony spicules through the sinus is almost diagnostic of chronic osteomyelitis

SKELETAL TUBERCULOSIS

TB spine:

- Most Common/Most common site of skeletal TB: Vertebrae
- Skeletal TB is the third most common type of tuberculosis (First is TB of lungs and second is TB of lymph nodes)
- Most common region involved in spinal TB: T9-L1 (Dorso-lumbar)
- Earliest symptom of spinal TB: Back Pain
- TB bacilli reach spine through hematogenous route (paravertebral plexus of Batson's)
- Most common subtype of spinal TB is paradiscal
- Infection reach spine because of some primary focus (lungs, lymph nodes)
- Healing of spinal TB occurs with bony ankylosis
- Pott's paraplegia refers to neurological complications commonly seen with thoracic spine TB where spinal cord is affected

TB Knee:

- Begins in synovium
- Long standing TB knee results in triple deformity (knee flexion, lateral rotation and posterior subluxation)

TB hip:

- Most commonly affects children
- Night cries: Because of relaxation of muscles at night, bony surfaces rub against each other producing severe pain
- Pain is referred to knee joint because of same nerve of hip and knee joint
- Fixed flexion deformity at hip is judged by Thomas test
- TB hip heals by fibrous ankylosis

VI. METABOLIC BONE DISORDERS

RICKETS

Pathology:

- Defective mineralization of osteoid/bones and cartilage because of relative or absolute deficiency of vitamin D
- Increased uncalcified osteoid in the immature skeletal framework

Features:

- Presents by 3 – 7 months of age

- Craniotabes (flattening of the occiput and accumulation of osteoid in the frontal and parietal regions)
- Wide open fontanelle
- Rachitic rosary (Cupping of anterior ends of ribs and enlargement of costochondral junction)
- Bowing of legs (genu varum or wind-swept deformity)
- Triradiate pelvis
- Harrison's sulcus (retraction of lower part of chest wall because of soft ribs)

X-ray appearances:

- Widening and thickening of epiphysis/growth plate
- Cupping, splaying and fraying of metaphysis is the earliest change seen at lower ends of radius and ulna

VII. ARTHRITIS

Rheumatoid arthritis:

- RA is a disease of: Synovium/synovial membrane
- There is hypertrophy of synovium with formation of granulation tissue over cartilage (pannus)
- RA is an autoimmune condition with inflammation of synovium/joint
- Associated with HLA-DR4
- There is symmetrical hypertrophy of small joints of hands (MCP and PIP, but never DIP)
- Patients come with the complaints of morning stiffness which gets better with exercise/movements
- Ulnar deviation of fingers may occur
- Most dangerous complication is atlanto-axial subluxation
- Managed by NSAIDs, steroids, DMARDS/disease modifying anti-rheumatoid drugs like methotrexate, chloroquine, sulfasalazine, gold salts etc.
- Mostly affects: Females (three times)

Ankylosing spondylitis/Marie Strumpell disease/Bechetrew disease:

- Associated HLA: HLA B27
- Enthesitis (point of attachment of tendons/cartilage to bone is painful)
- Enthesopathy (especially around pelvis and heel) Affects young adults
- Back-pain
- There is limitation of flexion and extension of lumbar spine
- Extra-articular manifestations include acute anterior uveitis (most common and occurs in about one-third cases of AS), inflammatory bowel disease etc
- X-ray shows: Bamboo spine
- Earliest radiological change is haziness of sacroiliac spine (sacroiliitis)

Osteoarthritis:

- Usually OA involves:
  - o Hip (in western world)
  - o Knee (in Indian setup)
- Does not affect MCP joint (which is most common joint affected in rheumatoid arthritis)
- Interphalangeal joints and nodes:
  - o DIP: Heberdens node
  - o PIP: Bouchard nodes
- Types:
  - o Primary:
    - – Most common type
    - – No known cause
  - o Secondary:
    - – Occurs because of mismanaged articular fractures, inflammatory arthropathy etc
- Clinical feature:
  - o Asymmetric arthritis (recall symmetric arthritis of rheumatoid arthritis)
  - o Joint crepitus
  - o Pain along joint line (initially with activity and but later on even at rest)
- Management:
  - o NSAIDs
  - o Intra-articular steroid injections
  - o For rest pain, arthroplasty (joint replacement)

For better preparation and success in AIIMS-NORCET Exam, download **'drkamalkvgroup'** mobile app from Google Playstore.

WhatsApp: +91 84 7000 4333

VIII. REGIONAL ORTHOPEDICS

CTEV:

- Manipulation should begin:
  - o Immediately after birth by mother after every feed
  - o This should be carried out for a month till the skin is mature enough to tolerate the cast
- Corrective manipulation and casting is done only after first month
- CTEV/clubfoot can be idiopathic or secondary
- Idiopathic CTEV: Present since birth and there is no definitive cause
- Clinical features:
  - o Size of foot and heel is small
  - o Deformities of foot are forefoot adduction, equinus, inversion, varus and tibial torsion
  - o Deep creases are noted on the medial side of sole and back of heel
  - o Lateral border of foot is gently convex
- Nowadays management is by serial casting by Ponseti technique

Carpal tunnel syndrome/CTS:

- CTS is because of compression of median nerve as it passes beneath the flexor retinaculum
- Causes of CTS (CARPAL-MD):
  - o **C**: Colle's fracture
  - o **A**: Acromegaly
  - o **R**: Rheumatoid arthritis
  - o **P**: Pregnancy
  - o **A**: Amyloidosis
  - o **L**: Low thyroid (hypothyroidism)
  - o **M**: Myxedema
  - o **D**: Dislocation of lunate bone
- Patient presents with complaints of tingling in the lateral two and a half fingers. Later on there may be wasting of thenar eminence and decreased sensation over lateral three and a half fingers on volar side
- Managed by either steroid injections or decompression surgery by dividing flexor retinaculum

IX. NERVE INJURIES

Terms/Fractures and Nerves involved:

- Meralgia paresthetica involves: Lateral cutaneous nerve of thigh
- Winging of scapula involves: Long thoracic nerve of Bell
- Foot drop: Common peroneal nerve (Related to neck of fibula)
- Supracondylar # humerus: Median nerve (Anterior interosseous nerve)
- Tarsal tunnel syndrome: Posterior tibial nerve entrapment

Ulnar nerve:

- Positive card test (weak palmar interossei; patient is unable to hold card between fingers)
- Ulnar claw hand (partial claw hand if only ulnar nerve is injured; total clawing is seen if both the ulnar and median nerves are injured)

Median nerve:

- Carpal tunnel syndrome
- Pointing index/Oschner's clasping test
- Ape thumb/simian deformity

Radial nerve:

- Saturday night palsy
- Crutch palsy
- Paralysis of radial nerve results in wrist drop (paralysis of extensors of wrists and fingers)

Axillary nerve:

- Injured in anterior dislocation of shoulder
- Fracture surgical neck of humerus
- Faulty intramuscular injections in deltoid

For better preparation and success in AIIMS-NORCET Exam, download **'drkamalkvgroup'** mobile app from Google Playstore.

WhatsApp: +91 84 7000 4333

SECTION 7: BASICS OF OPHTHALMOLOGY

I. OCULAR ANATOMY AND PHYSIOLOGY

APPENDAGES OF THE EYE

Conjunctiva:

- Epithelium (stratified squamous non-keratinized)
- Adenoid layer
- Fibrous layer

Glands of eyelids:

- Meibomian/tarsal glands
- Gland of Zeis
- Gland of Moll

Lacrimal apparatus:

- Lacrimal gland
- Lacrimal sac

Nasolacrimal duct:

- 12 – 24 mm long
- Runs downwards, slightly outwards and backwards
- Opens into inferior meatus of nose
- At lower end, valve of Hasner is present

EYEBALL

Dimensions:

- Total AP diameter/axial length: 24 mm
- Horizontal diameter: 23.5 mm
- Vertical diameter: 23 mm
- Depth of anterior chamber: 2-3 mm
- Circumference: 75 mm
- Volume: 6.5 cc
- Weight: 7 gm
- Length of optic nerve: 4.7-5 cm

Segments:

- Anterior (anterior and posterior chamber)
- Posterior

Anterior chamber:

- Depth: 2.5 – 3 mm
- Anterior to iris
- Shallower in hypermetropes
- Deeper in myopes

Anterior segment:

- Includes crystalline lens and structure anterior to it (cornea, iris, anterior and posterior chamber)

EXTRAOCULAR MUSCLES

Extraocular muscles:

- 4 recti arises from common tendinous ring (annulus of Zinn) at the apex of orbit, and are inserted onto the sclera
- SR and MR have an attachment with the dural sheath of the optic nerve (therefore painful movements in retrobulbar neuritis)
- IR is the only muscle arising from floor of the orbit. It is the shortest extraocular muscle
- SR is the longest extraocular muscle

NERVE SUPPLY

- 3rd cranial nerve: SR, MR, IR and IO
- 4th cranial nerve: SO
- 6th cranial nerve: LR

DEVELOPMENT

Eye in newborn:

- Orbit is more divergent (50 degree)
- Retina is fully developed (except macula)
- Cornea is relatively large (10 mm)
- Hypermetropia of +2.5D
- Visual acuity of 6/60

PHYSIOLOGY

Transparency of cornea:

- Peculiar arrangement of corneal lamellae
- Avascularity of cornea
- Swelling pressure of cornea
- Relative dehydration of cornea

Transparency of lens:

- Arrangement of lens proteins
- Avascularity of lens
- Tightly packed lens fibres
- Semi-permeable lens capsule
- Aquaporin-O

II. CLINICAL METHODS IN OPHTHALMOLOGY

OPHTHALMOLOGICAL TEST

Direct ophthalmoscopy:

- Image is virtual and erect
- Magnified 15 times in emmetropes (more in myopes and less in hypermetropes)

Indirect ophthalmoscopy:

- Image is real and inverted
- Magnified 5 times with +13D lens

Retinoscopy:

- Done with plane mirror
- Distance of 1 m

Other procedures:

- Keratometry: Measures curvature of cornea
- Retinoscopy: Objective assessment of refractive state of eye
- Gonioscopy: Measures angle of anterior chamber
- Ishihara plates, Hardy Rand Rittler plates: Color vision
- Landolt's rings: Visual acuity in children/illiterates
- Slit lamp examination: Best to demonstrate aqueous flare and keratic precipitates
- Campimetry/Scotometry: Performed to evaluate the central and paracentral area (30 degrees) of the visual field on Bjerrum's screen

Gonioscopy:

- Koeppe goniolens provides a direct view of the angle of anterior chamber

Tonometry:

- Measures intraocular pressure
- Schiotz tonometer is most commonly used (indentation tonometry)

Form sense:

- Snellen chart tests: Vision (measure of form sense)

Perimetry:

- Normal extent of field of vision
- Superior and Nasal: 60 degrees
- Inferior: 70 degrees
- Temporal: 90 degrees

For better preparation and success in AIIMS-NORCET Exam, download **'drkamalkvgroup'** mobile app from Google Playstore.

WhatsApp: +91 84 7000 4333

III. OCULAR PHARMACOLOGY

Anti-viral drugs:

- Acyclovir: Effective in most forms of herpes simplex and herpes zoster
- Ganciclovir: Used in CMV retinitis

Anti-fungal drugs:

- Amphotericin-B:
  - o Effective against candida, histoplasma and Cryptococcus
  - o Intravitreal injection for fungal endophthalmitis
- Ketoconazole: Single oral dose in fungal keratitis and endophthalmitis

Mydriatics:

- Shortest and quickly acting mydriatic: Tropicamide
- Mydriatic with no cycloplegia: Phenylephrine
- Mydriatic used as a ointment in children: Atropine

Lasers:

- Argon laser: Used in diabetic retinopathy
- Krypton laser: Used in peripheral retinal vascular abnormalities
- Diode: Used in intraocular tumours
- Nd:YAG: Used for capsulotomy and iridotomy
- Excimer: Used in refractive corneal surgery (LASIK)

ANTIGLAUCOMA DRUGS

Drugs increasing trabecular meshwork:

- Miotics (Pilocarpine)
- Epinephrine, Dipivefrine
- Bimatoprost

Drugs which increase uveoscleral outflow:

- Prostaglandin (Latanoprost)
- Epinephrine, Dipivefrine
- Brimonidine
- Apraclonidine

Drugs which decrease aqueous production:

- Carbonic anhydrase inhibitor (Acetazolamide, Dorzolamide)
- Alpha receptor stimulators in ciliary process (Epinephrine, Dipivefrine, Clonidine, Brimonidine, Apraclonidine)
- Beta blockers (Timolo, Betaxolol)

Hyperosmotic agents:

- Glycerol
- Mannitol

IV. DISEASES OF CONJUNCTIVA

CONJUNCTIVITIS

Spring catarrh/Vernal keratoconjunctivitis:

- Common in children/young adult (males 4-20 years)
- Type I hypersensitivity
- Palpebral form is most common than bulbar and mixed types
- Intense itching
- Mucoid stringy/ropy discharge known as Maxwell Lyon sign
- Horner Tranta's spots at limbus
- Cobblestone papillae on upper tarsal conjunctiva
- Alkaline tears
- Management: Mast cell stabilizers

TRACHOMA/EGYPTIAN OPHTHALMIA

Features:

- Caused by chlamydia trachomatis
- Serotypes A, B, Ba and C are associated with hyperendemic (blinding) trachoma
- Spreads by direct contact with fomites and flies
- Chlamydia trachomatis is epitheliotropic
- Produces intracytoplasmic inclusion bodies (Halberstaedter Prowazeke bodies)
- IP: 5-21 days
- Herbert's pits (scarred limbal follicles)
- Arlt's line (conjunctival scarring; upper tarsal conjunctiva)
- Follicles > 5 mm
- Entropion
- Trichiasis
- Pathognomonic features of trachoma follicles are presence of Leber cells and areas of necrosis

Management:

- Single oral dose of azithromycin/tetracycline ointment for 6 weeks
- DOC (locally): Tetracycline ointment
- SAFE strategy

SAFE strategy:

- Surgery
- Antibiotics
- Facial cleanliness
- Environmental improvement

V. DISEASES OF CORNEA

Anatomy:

- Epithelium: Non-keratinized stratified squamous
- Cornea can absorb oxygen from: Air (directly)
- Nutrients can diffuse into cornea from: Aqueous humour
- Refractive index: 1.33D
- Refractive power: 45D
- Endothelium is responsible for maintaining transparency of cornea

Size:

- Microcornea: <10 mm horizontal diameter (pthisis bulbi)
- Megalocornea: >13 mm (buphthalmos)

Keratoconus

- Protrusion of central part of cornea with thinning (conical shape)
- Munson's sign (localised bulging of lower lid when patient looks down; positive in late stages)
- Fleischer ring (Seen at the base of cone is due to hemosiderin deposition in epithelium)
- Bilateral in 85% cases
- Most common in girls after puberty

VI. GLAUCOMA

PRIMARY CONGENITAL GLAUCOMA

Presentation:

- 40% cases are present since birth (Newborn glaucoma/True congenital glaucoma)
- In 50%, manifests prior to the age of 2 years (Infantile glaucoma)
- In 10%, presents between 2-10 years (Juvenile glaucoma)
- AR inheritance
- Male: Female: 3:2
- Boys affected more
- Bilateral in 75% cases

Features:

- 1st symptom: Lacrimation
- Photophobia
- Occurs before the age of 3 characterized by enlarged eyeball, corneal diameter >13 mm
- Corneal edema (first sign)
- Haab's striae (healed splits in Descemet's membrane)
- Deep anterior chamber
- Raised IOP (intraocular pressure) and Variable optic cupping

Treatment:

- Goniotomy is the surgery of choice (80% success rate)
- Trabeculotomy (done when corneal couding prevents visualization of angle for goniotomy)
- Combined trabeculotomy and trabeculectomy is now-a-days the preferred surgery with better results

PRIMARY OPEN ANGLE GLAUCOMA/ POAG

Presentation:

- High myopes are predisposed
- >40 years

Pathology:

- There is increased resistance to outflow of the aqueous offered by:
    - o The sclerosed trabecular meshwork
    - o The scelrosed endothelium lining of the canal of Schlemm

Features:

- Mostly asymptomatic or, Progressive painless loss of vision
- Usually noticed when vision is completely lost in one eye and the other eye is seriously impaired
- Reading or close work is often difficult due to accommodative failure
- There is frequent increase in the strength of presbyopic glasses
- Initially there is exaggeration of normal diurnal variation (>6 mm Hg is suspicious and >8 mm Hg is diagnostic)
- In later stages, IOP is permanently elevated (30-45 mm Hg)

Established POAG:

- IOP >23 mm Hg associated with definite disc cupping and visual field defects
- Established POAG (Triad):

- IOP: >23 mm Hg
- Disc cupping: +nt
- Visual field defects: +nt

Glaucoma suspect/ocular hypertension:

- IOP: >23 mm Hg
- Disc cupping: Absent (-nt)
- Visual field defects: -nt

Low tension/Normal tension glaucoma:

- IOP: <21 mm Hg
- Disc cupping: +nt (Present)
- Visual field defects: +nt

Treatment:

- Medical: Treatment of choice
- Surgical: Last resort
- Argon Laser trabeculoplasty

Medical treatment:

- Local: Pilocarpine, Timolol, Betaxalol, Epinephrine
- 1st line of treatment: Timolol (beta blocker)/Pilocarpine
- Systemic: Acetazolamide
- Hyperosmotic agents: Glycerol (oral), Mannitol (I/V)

Surgical treatment:

- Trabeculectomy
- Argon laser trabeculoplasty: Causes shrinkage of the collagen on the inner surface of the trabecular ring, thereby opening the intertrabecular spaces

PRIMARY ANGLE CLOSURE GLAUCOMA/ PACG

Predisposing factors:

- Hypermetropes with shallow anterior chamber
- Eye in which iris-lens diaphragm is placed anteriorly
- Male: Female: 1:3
- Precipitating factors: Dim illuminations, emotional stress and use of mydriatics

Stages:

- Prodromal
- Phase of constant instability
- Stage of acute congestive attack
- Stage of chronic closed angle glaucoma
- Absolute glaucoma

Treatment:

- Medical
- Surgical

Medical:

- Local: Pilocarpine/timolol/betaxalol
- Systemic: Acetazolamide/sedative
- Hyperosmotic: Glycerol (oral), mannitol (I/V)

Surgical:

- Always indicated for permanent cure
- But lower the IOP by drugs before surgery
- Laser iridotomy
- Peripheral iridectomy
- Trabeculectomy, in case of extensive peripheral synechiae

VII. DISEASES OF THE LENS

Anatomy:

- Lens derives its nutrition from: Aqueous humour
- Lens is thicker: Anteriorly

CATARACT

Types:

- Congenital/Developmental
- Acquired

Congenital cataract:

- Punctate
- Zonular
- Coronary
- Anterior capsular
- Posterior capsular

Acquired cataract:

- Senile
- Cataract associated with ocular diseases
- Cataract associated with systemic diseases
- Traumatic cataract
- After cataract

SENILE CORTICAL CATARACT

Stages:

- Immature: Lamellar separation, Incipient, Intumescent
- Mature
- Hypermature

Mature cataract:

- Entire cortex is opaque
- Iris shadow is absent

Hypermature/Morgagnian cataract:

- Cortex becomes fluid and appears milky
- Nucleus sinks by gravity in the bag of liquefied cortex
- Iridodonesis (tremulousness of iris)
- Deep anterior chamber

Early symptoms of acquired cataract:

- Black dots
- Uniocular polyopia
- Coloured halos

Late symptoms:

- Vision improves in bright light in peripheral opacity
- Vision improves in dim light in central opacity
- Visual loss is out of proportion to the size of opacity in posterior cortical cataract
- There is progressive myopia so that a presbyopic person gets "second sight" or "improvement" in vision without glasses in nuclear sclerosis
- Vision is grossly reduced in mature cataract, reduced to counting fingers at few cms

Management of cataract:

- ICCE
- ECCE
- Phacoemulsification
- Manual small incision cataract surgery/SICS

Intracapsular lens extraction:

- Entire lens along with the capsule is removed by intracapsular forceps or cryoprobe
- Indicated in subluxated/dislocated lens (suspensory ligament/ zonules broken)

Extracapsular lens extraction:

- Posterior capsule and posterior part of the anterior capsule are left behind after ECCE
- Posterior chamber IOL implant is gently inserted
- Indicated in <45 years (zonules are strong)
- IOL implant

Phacoemulsification:

- Nucleus is emulsified by the phacoemulsifier titanium probe
- All the lens matter is removed
- A small in the bag IOL or foldable soft silicone/hydrogen PHEMA (polyhydroxyethyl methacrylate) IOL is inserted

VIII. DISEASES OF THE RETINA

Diabetic retinopathy:

- Fundus examination in IDDM: 5 years after diagnosis of DM
- Fundus examination in NIDDM: As early as possible
- Relationship of diabetic retinopathy with disease duration: Incidence of diabetic retinopathy increases with disease duration

HIV:

- Most common abnormal finding on fundoscopic examination: Cotton-wool spots
- Most devastating consequences of HIV infection on eye: CMV retinitis

RETINAL DETACHMENT/RD

Definition:

- Separation of neurosensory retina (retina proper) from pigmentary epithelium by the subretinal fluid

Types:

- Primary/Simple/Rhegmatogenous (Myopia)
- Secondary/Non-rhegmatogenous

Primary RD:

- Always due to a break in the retina in the form of a hole/tear, which allows vitreous to seep through and raise the retina from its bed

Secondary RD:

- Always secondary to the ocular diseases/pathology

Treatment:

- Approximate and adhere the torn part of the retina to the choroid by:
  - o Photocoagulation
  - o Cryopexy
  - o Scleral buckling
  - o Pars plana vitrectomy

IX. TUMOURS OF THE EYE

RETINOBLASTOMA/RB

Features:

- Most common primary intraocular malignancy of childhood
- Hypothesis: Knudson's two stage hypothesis
- Inheritance: Autosomal dominant
- May be bilateral in: 30-40% cases (particularly familial ones)

Management:

- Chemotherapy for bilateral Rb or metastasis in Rb
- Enucleation for uniocular disease (advanced)

X. NEURO-OPHTHALMOLOGY

Anatomy:

- Most sensitive part of eye: Fovea (contains cones only)
- Fundus examination:
  - o Macula: 3 mm lateral to optic disc (cones > rods)
  - o Fovea: Centre of macula (only cones); maximum visual acuity
  - o Optic cup: Depressed area of optic disc (no rods or cones); physiological blind spot

Visual field defects:

- Homonymous hemianopia: Lesions of optic tract
- Superior Homonymous quadrantanopia: Lesion of temporal lobe
- Inferior/lower quadrantanopia is because of lesion in parietal lobe
- Bitemporal hemianopia: Lesions of optic chiasm

CRANIAL NERVES

3rd cranial nerve:

- Supplies all extraocular muscle EXCEPT Superior oblique and lateral rectus

4th cranial nerve:

- Weakness/paralysis of superior oblique muscle; which normally moves the eye downwards and inwards

6th cranial nerve:

- Weakness/paralysis of lateral rectus; which normally rotates the eye laterally

XI. DISEASES OF THE UVEAL TRACT

ACUTE ANTERIOR UVEITIS

Iridocyclitis:

- Most common in developing countries is hypersensitivity to tubercular proteins

HLA associated uveitis:

- HLA B27: Acute anterior uveitis associated with ankylosing spondylitis and Reiter's syndrome
- HLA B5: Behcet's disease

Treatment:

- Atropine is the most important drug in managing a case of acute iridocyclitis
- Steroids are effective in most of the cases

XII. OCULAR TRAUMA

Sympathetic ophthalmitis/SO:

- Region involved: Ciliary body is injured
- Mode of injury: Penetrating injury in ciliary region (dangerous region)
- 1st sign of SO: Keratic precipitates/Retrolental flare

Blow-out fracture of orbit:

- Most commonly involves the floor of orbit along the bone covering the infraorbital canal
- Double diplopia: Diplopia in both up and down gaze
- Infraorbital nerve anesthesia
- Enophthalmos (with severe fracture)
- Periocular ecchymosis
- Investigation:
  - o Water's X-ray view (tear drop sign)
  - o CT scan

XIII. DISEASES OF THE EYELID

Chalazion:

- Painless
- Chronic lipogranulomatous inflammation of Meibomian gland
- Recurrent chalazion may predispose to Adenocarcinoma of Meibomian gland

Internal hordeolum:

- Suppurative acute inflammation of meibomian gland

External hordeolum/stye:

- Painful
- Due to staphylococcus
- Suppurative inflammation of Zeis/Moll gland

Ptosis:

- Ptosis is drooping of Upper eyelid

XIV. REFRACTIVE ERRORS

Presbyopia:

- Physiological insufficiency of accommodation
- Due to loss of elasticity of lens capsule
- Treatment: Convex lens

Astigmatism:

- Spherical aberration
- Due to irregular curvature of cornea
- Cornea curved differently in different meridians

Aphakia:

- Absence of natural crystalline lens from its position as after surgery, posterior dislocation
- Deep anterior chamber
- Jet black pupil
- Iridodonesis
- Management is PCIOL

MYOPIA

Features:

- Distant vision is defective

- Children squeezes eye frequently
- Eyeball is large
- In pathological myopia, power increases even after 21 years
- Complications: Primary open angle glaucoma, retinal detachment
- Rays of light are focused: Front of retina
- Size of eyeball: Big

Management/Surgical procedure:

- Radial keratotomy (small degree; not done now a days): 1-6D
- Soft lens (any range)
- LASIK (laser assisted in situ keratomileusis): 2-12D

XV. DISEASES OF THE OPTIC NERVE

PAPILLOEDEMA

Seen in:

- Raised intracranial tension (intracranial infections like cavernous sinus thrombosis, cerebral abscess, brain tumours/ intracranial space occupying lesions)

Management:

- Treat the underlying cause of raised intracranial pressure

PAPILLITIS/OPTIC NEURITIS

Features:

- Unilateral
- Marked loss of vision
- Tenderness at the insertion of muscles
- Central/centrocaecal scotoma
- Most common cause: Multiple sclerosis
- Pseudopapillitis is seen in: Hypermetropia

Management:

- Methyl prednisolone

XVI. EYE IN SYSTEMIC DISEASES

Hyperthyroidism:

- Lid lag (Von Grafes sign)
- Poor convergence (Mobius sign)
- External ophthalmoplegia
- Large extraocular muscles
- Muscle most commonly involved in thyroid ophthalmopathy: Inferior rectus

XVII. BLINDNESS

Facts:

- Most common cause of ocular morbidity in India: Refractive error
- Most common cause of blindness in children in India: Vitamin A deficiency
- Most common cause of blindness in adults in India: Cataract

SECTION 8: BASICS OF DERMATOLOGY

I. ANATOMY AND PHYSIOLOGY

Anatomy:

- Skin/epidermis epithelium: Keratinized, stratified squamous
- Normal turn over time of epidermis/Skin doubling time is: 4 weeks

Structure of skin:

- Epidermis
- Dermis
- Subcutaneous fatty tissue

Layers of epidermis:

- Basal cell layer/Stratum basale/stratum germinativum:
  - o Mitotically active
  - o Contains melanocytes and Merkel cells (mechanoreceptors)
- Prickle cell layer/Stratum spinosum
- Granular cell layer/Stratum granulosus
- Transitional cell layer/Stratum lucidum: Seen only in skin of palms and soles
- Horny cell layer/Stratum corneum: Provides mechanical protection and acts as a barrier to water loss

II. VENEREAL DISEASES

Chancroid:

- Chancroid/soft sore/soft chancre: H. ducreyi
- Painful, irregular, non-indurated, genital ulcers
- Suppuration of regional lymph nodes (inflammatory bubo)
- Treatment: Azithromycin/ceftriaxone/ciprofloxacin/erythromycin

LGV:

- LGV/LGI is caused by: Chlamydia trachomatis (Most common by serotype L2)
- Characterized by involvement of lymphatic system
- Regional lymph node enlargement (climatic bubo)
- Glands are hard, tender, matted together
- Treatment: Doxycycline/Erythromycin/tetracycline

Granuloma inguinale:

- Donovanosis/Granuloma Inguinale/Granuloma venerum is caused by: Calymmatobacter/Klebsiella granulomatosis
- Chronic granulomatous and ulcerative infection of genitalia and surrounding skin
- Elevated, rounded, velvetty and granulomatous ulcer
- Treatment: Azithromycin/Cotrimoxazole

SYPHILIS/THE GREAT IMITATOR

Pathology:

- Caused by a spirochaete T. pallidum
- Dark ground microscope: Used to study morphology and motility of T. pallidum

Stages:

- Primary: Hunterian chancre (over penis/scrotum in males and vulva/cervix/perineum in females)
- Chancre is single, painless, ulcerated, indurated and highly infectious
- Associated with painless enlargement of regional lymph nodes

REITER'S SYNDROME

Features of Reiter's Syndrome:

- Urethritis (nonspecific urogenital infection)
- Bilateral conjunctivitis (30-50%) and anterior uveitis (4-5%)
- Arthritis (acute ascending asymmetric oligoarthritis)
- Nonsuppurative, monoarthritis or asymmetric oligoarthritis affectiing mainly knees, ankles and metatarsal joints

- Enthesitis
- Backache

III. DISORDERS OF SKIN APPENDAGES

Nails in dermatology:

- Mees line: Arsenic poisoning
- Koilonychia:
  - o Iron deficiency anemia
  - o Spoon shaped depression of the nail plate
- Onycholysis (separation of nail from bed):
  - o Psoriasis
  - o Fungal infection
  - o Trauma
- Koenen's periungual fibroma: Tuberous sclerosis

Acne vulgaris:

- Structure involved: Pilosebaceous glands
- Comedo/blackhead, seen in acne are:
  - o Small cysts, formed in hair follicles
  - o Overproduction of sebum and sebaceous duct blockage – the black top is because of melanin
- Topical agents for treatment:
  - o Retinoic acid
  - o Benzoyl peroxide
  - o Salicylic acid
- Oral treatment: Doxycyline/minocycline/erythromycin
- Severe nodulocystic acne not responsive to oral antibiotics, Hormonal therapy and Topical therapy requires: Synthetic retinoid/Isotretinoin (It is teratogenic)

Alopecia areata:

- Etiology of Alopecia areata:
  - o Autoimmune
  - o T-cell mediated autoimmune condition that occurs in genetically predisposed patients
- Characteristic appearance of hair:
  - o Exclamation mark hair (stumps of hair)
  - o During the active stage of hair loss, broken off hair of 3-4 mm long, which tapers off towards the scalp are seen (exclamation mark hair)
- Recurrent, non-scarring alopecia
- Most commonly affected region is scalp
- There is well-circumscribed circular areas of hair-loss (2-6 mm in diameter)
- Associated features: Pitting of nails (Most common nail finding in alopecia areata)
- Treatment of alopecia areata: Minoxidil (Testosterone is contraindicated)

Other types of alopecia:

- Alopecia totalis: 100% hair loss over scalp
- Alopecia universalis: Complete loss of hairs on all hair-bearing areas of the body

IV. INFESTATIONS OF SKIN

Scabies:

- Incubation period: 4 weeks
- Pathognomic lesion of scabies: Burrows
- Location of burrow (layer of skin): Stratum corneum
- It takes about 3-4 weeks for itching to manifest after the infection is acquired
- Itching is worse at night when patient is warm and is off from his duties
- Burrows are slightly raised and brownish dark tortuous lines 1-10 mm in length
- Wrists, sides of fingers, webs spaces, genitalia and instep of foot are common sites
- Drug used orally for scabies: Ivermectin
- But DOC is 5% Permethrin

Pediculosis corporis:

- Vagabond's disease: Pediculosis corporis (body)

- Usually an outcome of poverty and unhygienic conditions where individuals rarely change their clothing
- In person harboring clothing lice for long periods of time, skin often becomes hyperpigmented (Vagabonds disease)
- Since lice completes its life cycle in clothing and not on the skin, treatment of pediculosis corporis is the treatment of clothing where the lice harbor

V. PAPULOSQUAMOUS DISORDERS

PSORIASIS

Features:

- Bimodal distribution (early peak at 16-22 years and late peak at 57-60 years)
- Morphology: Well defined, erythematous raised plaques with white scaling
- On further removal of the scale, a smooth glossy red membrane (Burkley's membrane) appears

Nail changes in psoriasis:

- Coarse pitting
- Onycholysis (separation of distal part of nail plate from nail bed)
- Rounded areas of discoloration of nail bed may look like an oil drop, below nail plate

Clinical diagnosis:

- Deep red colored well-defined plaques having easily removable silvery white scales
- Involvement of extensors
- Presence of nail changes

Photochemotherapy/PUVA-therapy:

- Psoralen + UV-A
- Minimal side-effects
- Psoralen are given orally on alternate days 2 hours before UV exposure
- Lesions usually clear in 1-2 months

LICHEN PLANUS

Features:

- Common sites are inner aspects of ankle and wrists, flexor aspect of forearm
- Wickham's striae: Fine network of gray/white lines of the lesions
- Civatte bodies (basal cell degeneration form 'colloid' or Civatte bodies in the epidermis)
- Basal cell liquefactive degeneration
- Koebner's phenomenon
- Nail changes: Nail plate thinning, onycholysis, pterygium
- Treatment: Spontaneous resolution in 6 months – 2 years
- Topical glucocorticoids
- Oral lichen planus is difficult to treat

5Ps of lichen planus:

- Pruritic
- Polygonal
- Purple (violaceous)
- Plain (flat topped)
- Papule/plaques

For better preparation and success in AIIMS-NORCET Exam, download **'drkamalkvgroup'** mobile app from Google Playstore.

WhatsApp: +91 84 7000 4333

VI. VESICOBULLOUS DISORDERS

Pemphigus:

- Most common form of pemphigus: P. vulgaris
- Intraepidermal (flaccid)
- Suprabasal Acantholytic bullae
- Blisters rupture easily leaving behind denuded skin
- Oral mucosal lesion (90%)
- Lesion heal without scarring
- Nikolsky sign is positive
- Definitive diagnosis of pemphigus: Demonstration of Anti-desmoglein autoantibodies by Direct immunofluorescence on Skin biopsy

Pemphigoid:

- Tense subepidermal bullae (in superficial layers/subcorneal) are seen in Pemphigoid
- Bullae are seen on flexor surfaces
- Direct immunofluorescence microscopy of the normal appearing perilesional skin shows linear deposits of IgG and/or C3

Dermatitis herpetiformis:

- Extremely itchy small papules and vesicles on knees and elbows (extensor surfaces)
- Subepidermal blister with neutrophils in the dermal papillae
- DH is associated with (almost in all patients): Gluten sensitive enteropathy (subclinical/asymptomatic)
- DOC for DH: Dapsone
- Also strictly exclude gluten from the diet

VII. INFECTIONS OF SKIN

HIV:

- Leads to reactivation of herpes zoster/shingles
- Shingles is characterized by unilateral vesicular eruption within a dermatome, often associated with severe pain
- Most commonly dermatomes involved are between T3-L3

Tinea:

- Athlete's foot/Tinea pedis presents as:
  - o Severe itching
  - o Hyperhydrosis (Does not affect only athletes)
  - o Most common dermatophytosis
  - o Caused by T. rubrum/T. mentgrophytes
- Onychomycosis/Tinea unguium/Ringworm of the nail affects: Nail plate
- Dhobi itch or jock itch is also known as: Tinea cruris

LEPROSY

Important points:

- Associated cells in lepromatous leprosy: Virchow cells/lepra cells (foamy macrophages laden with acid-fast bacilli)
- Virchow cells are seen in: Lepromatous leprosy
- Most common nerve involved: Ulnar nerve
- Organs not involved in leprosy (M. leprae grows better in cooler places):
  - o Warmer areas of skin and internal organs:
    - – Axilla
    - – Groin
    - – Scalp
    - – Midline back
    - – Ovaries
    - – Lung
    - – CNS
- Most common type of leprosy in India: TT

Management:

- 1st line of drugs:
  - o Rifampicin
  - o Clofazimine
  - o Dapsone
- Multibacillary leprosy:
  - o Rifampicin 600 mg once monthly supervised
  - o Dapsone 100 mg/day, unsupervised
  - o Clofazimine 300 mg once monthly supervised
- Paucibacillary leprosy:
  - o Rifampicin 600 mg once monthly supervised
  - o Dapsone 100 mg/day, unsupervised
- DOC in neuritis: Steroids
- Treatment of nerve abscess: Incision and drainage (Nerve abscess is most common in borderline tuberculoid leprosy)

Tuberculoid leprosy:

- Raised cell mediated immunity
- Lepromin test is positive (bacillary load is low)
- Microscopy: Non-caseating granuloma with epitheloid and giant cells

Lepromatous leprosy:

- Infective form of leprosy: Lepromatous leprosy
- Features of lepromatous leprosy:
  - o Gynaecomastia (because of testicular involvement)
  - o Madarosis (loss of eyebrows and eyelashes)
  - o Collapse of nasal bridge
  - o Leonine facies

- Decreased CMI/Cell mediated immunity
- High bacterial load (negative lepromin test)
- Symmetric, poorly marginated, multiple infiltrated nodules and plaques are seen

Lepra reaction seen in lepromatous leprosy:

- Type 1 (reversal reaction)
- Type 2 (erythema nodosum leprosum)

Lepromin test:

- Lepromin test indicates: Strong immunity
- It is a useful tool for evaluating the cell mediated immunity/ immune status of leprosy patients
- Lepromin test is not diagnostic
- It is helpful in estimating prognosis in leprosy of all varieties

TB SKIN

Lupus vulgaris:

- Lupus vulgaris is: Skin TB with no underlying active focus in the lung/lymph nodes
- Most common form of skin TB
- Most common in females
- Most common in head-neck region
- Red-brown plaques
- On diascopy, shows 'apple jelly nodules'

Scrofuloderma:

- Skin TB secondary to involvement of underlying structure i.e. joint, lymph node is: Scrofuloderma
- Results because of direct extension from underlying focus like infected lymph nodes, bones or muscles
- Firm, painless and subcutaneous nodules which suppurate to form ulcers with undermined edges and sinus tracts

Dermatological conditions caused by staphylococcus:

- SSSS (Staphylococcal scalded skin syndrome)
- Bullous impetigo/Impetigo contagiosa
- Furuncles/Boils
- Sycosis barbae and Sycosis nuchae

Bullous impetigo:

- Caused by coagulase positive Staph aureus
- Seen in neonates
- Thick walled persistent blisters on bland skin
- Can lead to SSSS, cellulitis

Non-bullous imetigo/impetigo contagiosa:

- Caused by GABHS (group A beta-hemolytic streptococci) and staph aureus
- Seen in children
- Thin walled blisters on erythematous base which ruptures leaving behind 'honey-coloured crusts'

VIII. ECZEMA

Atopic dermatitis:

- Face and trunk is involved in infants
- Positive family history of atopic triad (Allergic rhinitis, dermatitis and asthma)
- Also known as: Itch disease
- The cardinal symptom is pruritis and scratching may account for most of the signs
- Dennie-Morgan line/atopic pleat (An extra-fold of skin that develops under the eye)
- Increased palmar markings (hyperlinear palms)
- Increased number of skin creases on the palms
- Best test to diagnose AD: Clinical evaluation

For better preparation and success in AIIMS-NORCET Exam, download **'drkamalkvgroup'** mobile app from Google Playstore.

WhatsApp: +91 84 7000 4333

IX. PITYRIASIS

Pityriasis rosea:

- Herald/mother patch (solitary, salmon-pink, annular plaque, 2-6 cm in diameter, usually on the trunk)
- Cigarette paper scales (delicate peripheral scale)
- Christmas tree distribution: Lesions on the back are parallel to the ribs
- Treatment:
  - o Self limiting in 4-10 weeks

- o Oral antihistamines and topical glucocorticoids for itching

Pityriasis versicolor/tinea versicolor/versatile colour:

- Caused by (versi means several): Malassezia furfur (hyphal form) a dimorphic, lipophilic organism)
- Ovary, scaly macules and patches on the chest, shoulders and back
- Diagnosis: KOH preparations of scaling lesion shows 'spaghetti and meatballs' appearance
- Treatment: Selenium sulfide 2.5% shampoo/topical imidazole antifungals

X. SKIN TUMOURS

Mycosis fungoides:

- Cutaneous T cell lymphoma
- Most common skin lymphoma (CTCL/cutaneous T-cell lymphoma)
- Extranodal, indolent Non-Hodgkin Lymphoma that primarily develops on skin, but can involve the lymph nodes, blood and visceral organs
- Affects males in 6th decade

Acanthosis nigricans:

- Dark, Thick, Velvetty skin (in body folds and creases)
- Prominent on the dorsum of the neck and major flexures (axillae/groin)
- Most common endocrinal cause of acanthosis nigricans: Type 2 DM (otherwise most common association is with obesity)
- Also associated with acromegaly, Cushing's syndrome, PCOD etc.
- Internal malignancies associated with acanthosis nigricans:
  - o Adenocarcinoma lungs
  - o Gastric adenocarcinoma

BASAL CELL CA

Features:

- Spread of Basal cell Ca: Direct
- BCC does not show lymphatic spread
- Malignant epithelial tumour of basal cells
- Locally invasive
- Rarely metastasize

Treatment:

- Excision with margin examination
- Mohs micrographic surgery (MMS)

XI. MISCELLANEOUS CONDITIONS

Wood's lamp:

- Light generated in Wood's lamp: 360 nm ultraviolet/black light
- Wood's lamp filter is made of: Nickel and silica
- Appearance of erythrasma in Wood's lamp: Coral red colour

TUBEROUS SCLEROSIS

Ash leaf spot:

- White-ovoid macules of 1-3 cm size: Commonly seen over trunk and limbs
- Earliest manifestation

Adenoma sebaceum/angiofibromas:

- Consists of hyperplastic blood vessels and sebaceous glands
- Nasolabial folds, cheeks and chin are preferred sites

Shagreen patches:

- Seen in lumbosacral region as 1-10 cm size
- Slightly elevated, skin colored, soft irregularly thickened plaque giving an 'orange peel' or 'elephant hide' appearance

SECTION 9: BASICS OF E.N.T.

I. EAR

Parts:

- Outer: Transmits sound to inner ear
- Middle: Transmits sound to inner ear
- Inner: Converts sound to fluid motion and later on to electrical impulses

EXTERNAL EAR

External auditory canal:

- External ear contains:
  - o Pinna (contains elastic cartilage)
  - o External auditory canal
- Nerve supply of external auditory canal:
  - o Anterior wall and roof: Auriculotemporal nerve
  - o Posterior wall and floor: Vagus (auricular branch)
- Length of external auditory canal/EAC: 24 mm
- EAC is cartilaginous in: Outer third
- EAC is bony in: Inner two-thirds

Tympanic membrane:

- Parts of tympanic membrane:
  - o Pars tensa
  - o Pars flaccida (Shrapnel's membrane)
- Pars tensa:
  - o Forms most of TM
  - o Annulus tympanicus at periphery
  - o Central part is tented inwards at the level of tip of malleus (umbo)
  - o Bright cone of light radiating from the tip of malleus
- Normal appearance of tympanic membrane: Pearly white
- Surface area of tympanic membrane:
  - o Total: 90 mm^2
  - o Functional: 55 mm^2
- Partition between the EAC and middle ear
- Obliquely set
- Posterosuperior part if more lateral than its anteroinferior part
- 9 mm tall
- 9 mm wide
- 0.1 mm thick
- Layers of TM:
  - o 3 layers
  - o Outer epithelial layer
  - o Inner mucosal layer
  - o Middle fibrous layer

MIDDLE EAR

Middle ear cleft/MEC:

- Middle ear cleft: Mastoid air cells + mastoid antrum + aditus + attic + middle ear + eustachian tube
- MEC is lined by mucous membrane and filled with air

ME is divided into:

- Mesotympanum
- Epitympanum/attic
- Hypotympanum

Walls of ME:

- ME is a 6 sided box with roof, floor, 4 walls (medial, lateral, anterior and posterior)

Mastoid antrum:

- Large, air-containing space in the upper part of mastoid
- Communicates with attic through aditus
- Roof is formed by tegmen atri
- Lateral wall is formed by a plate of bone (suprameatal triangle)

Ossicles of ME:

- Malleus
- Incus
- Stapes
- Ossicles conduct sound energy from the tympanic membrane to the oval window and then to the inner ear fluid

Intratympanic muscles:

- Tensor tympani
- Stapedius

INNER EAR

Internal ear/Labyrinth:

- Important organ for hearing and balance
- Consists of bony and a membranous labyrinth
- Membranous labyrinth is filled with a clear fluid called endolymph
- Space between the bony and the membranous labyrinth is filled with perilymph

Bony labyrinth:

- Has 3 parts: the vestibule, the semicircular canals (SCC) and the cochlea

Membranous labyrinth:

- Consists of the cochlear duct, the utricle and the saccule, the 3 semicircular ducts, and the endolymphatic duct and sac

Important points:

- Location of inner ear: Petrous part of temporal bone
- Nerve which gets injured in inner ear (transverse fractures of temporal bone): Facial nerve
- Location of organ of Corti: Organ of Corti (with its hair cells) rests on Basilar membrane
- Content of perilymph:
  - o Resemble ECF
  - o Low K^+ and high Na^+
- Angular acceleration is sensed by: Semi-circular canal

For better preparation and success in AIIMS-NORCET Exam, download **'drkamalkvgroup'** mobile app from Google Playstore.

WhatsApp: +91 84 7000 4333

EUSTACHIAN TUBE

Eustachian tube:

- 3-3.8 cm in length
- Lateral 1/3rd bony
- Medial 2/3rd is cartilaginous
- Runs forwards, downwards and medially
- Shorter, wider and more horizontal in children
- Development of eustachian tube: 1st pharyngeal pouch
- Special feature of eustachian tube: Opens during swallowing (Tensor palati)

For better preparation and success in AIIMS-NORCET Exam, download **'drkamalkvgroup'** mobile app from Google Playstore.

WhatsApp: +91 84 7000 4333

TUNING FORK TEST

Rinne's test:

- Performed for: Detecting type and degree of deafness
- Procedure:
  - o Air conduction/AC is compared with bone conduction/ BC
  - o In normal subject, AC > BC
- Positive (AC > BC) test suggest:
  - o Normal
  - o Sensorineural hearing loss
- Negative test (BC > AC) suggest: Conductive deafness

Weber's test:

- Performed: With 512 Hz frequency tuning fork
- Procedure:
  - o Base of vibrating tuning fork is placed on the patient's forehead
  - o He had to note sound is equal in both ears or better in any

- o Normally a normal patient should hear equally in both the ears
- Conductive deafness: Sound is lateralized to diseased ear
  - o Suppose if a patient comes to you with reduced hearing in right ear. In Weber test, patient says that he feel sound is going toward right ear. It means he is having conductive type of deafness in right ear.
  - o Rinne's test should also be done
- Sensorineural deafness: Sound is lateralized to normal ear
  - o Suppose if a patient comes to you with reduced hearing in right ear. In Weber test, patient says that he feel sound is going toward left ear. It means he is having sensorineural type of deafness in right ear
  - o Rinne's test should also be done

DISEASES OF EXTERNAL EAR

Cauliflower ear:

- Haematoma of auricle (due to repeated trauma in Boxers and wrestlers)
- Infection of haematoma may result in perichondritis (usually by Pseudomonas)

Malignant otitis externa:

- Infection with P. aeruginosa
- Elderly diabetics with poor metabolic control (uncontrolled diabetes) or immunocompromised patients
- Feature: Dark ear discharge
- Management: Systemic antibiotics, aural toilet

DISEASES OF MIDDLE EAR

Secretory otitis media/Glue ear/Otitis media with effusion:

- Dysfunction of eustachian tube (nasopharyngitis, adnoid hyperplasia) resulting in fluid collection in middle ear
- Minimal/absent pain
- Sense of fullness in ear
- Hearing loss (inattentive behaviour)
- Medical treatment ineffective
- Myringotomy with Ventilation tube (grommet) insertion/ myringotomy with adenoidectomy

Otosclerosis:

- Most common cause of non-suppurative conductive deafness in adult males
- Common in Indians and Whites
- Most common in males (in India)
- Most common in females (Worldwide)
- 15-36 year age group
- May be aggravated by pregnancy
- Normal intact and freely mobile eardrum
- Most common site of otosclerosis:
  - o Oval window
  - o There is vascular spongy bone formation near the oval window resulting in ankylosis/fixation of stapes footplate
- Most common bone affected in otosclerosis: Stapes
- Type of deafness in otosclerosis: Progressive conductive deafness, usually bilateral
- Family history:
  - o Positive in 70% of cases
  - o Autosomal dominant
- Surgery of choice for otosclerosis: Stapedectomy (stapes including its footplate) + artificial prosthesis (Surgery of choice)
- Drug which can retard the progression: Sodium fluoride for cochlear otosclerosis

CHRONIC SUPPURATIVE OTITIS MEDIA

Features:

- Pathology: Basically a bony erosion
- Location (Bone): Usually found in apex of petrous temporal bone
- Associated perforation: Attic/posterior-superior marginal region is usually involved

Types of CSOM:

- Safe
- Unsafe

Management of CSOM:

- Modified radical mastoidectomy is done (spares the tympanic membrane and ossicles)

DISEASES OF THE INNER EAR

Meniere's disease:

- Disorder of inner ear where there is dilatation of endolymphatic sac.
- Increased endolymph secretion
- Affects scala media (cochlear duct) and saccule
- Associated with syphilis
- Most common in males
- Affects 35-60 years
- Unilateral
- Sense of fullness/pressure in ear
- Triad of Meniere's disease:
  - o Unilateral fluctuating/episodic hearing loss (low frequency sensorineural)
  - o Tinnitus (non pulsatile)
  - o Recurrent episodic prostrating vertigo
- Management:
  - o Vasodilators
  - o Surgery (stellate ganglion block, vestibule neurectomy)
  - o Decompression

Bells palsy:

- Unilateral facial palsy
- Lower motor neuron lesion
- Acute onset
- Increased predisposition in DM

Acoustic neurinoma/Vestibular schwannoma:

- Most common cerebellopontine angle tumour
- Affects 40-60 years
- Bilateral acoustic neuromas are associated with neurofibromatosis –II (central type)
- Hypoesthesia of posterior meatal wall (Hitzeliberger's sign)
- They arise from: Vestibular division of the eight nerve
- Benign tumour from neurilemmal sheath
- Most commonly involved structure: Superior vestibular nerve
- Earliest symptom: Unilateral progressive sensorineural deafness with tinnitus
- Loss of corneal reflex (earliest sign)
- Difficulty in balancing
- Surgery/Stereotactic surgery

II. NOSE

Function of nose:

- Respiration
- Humidification
- Olfaction
- Dust filtration

ANATOMY OF NOSE

Roof of nose:

- Cribriform plate of ethmoid

Nasal septum:

- 3 layers
- Septum proper in middle
- Mucoperichondrial lining on either side
- Septum is mainly formed by perpendicular plate of ethmoid, spine of maxilla, spine of palatine and vomer

Lateral wall of nose:

- 3 turbinates/conchae
- Superior and middle concha are part of ethmoid bone
- Inferior concha is a separate bone

Paranasal air sinuses:

- Maxillary

- Ethmoid
- Frontal
- Sphenoid

Meatus and openings:

- Sphenoethmoidal recess: Sphenoid sinus
- Superior meatus: Posterior ethmoid sinus
- Middle meatus:
  - o Frontal sinus
  - o Maxillary sinus (at hiatus semilunaris)
  - o Anterior and middle ethmoidal
- Inferior meatus: Nasolacrimal duct

DISEASES OF THE NOSE

Depressed nasal bridge/saddle nose:

- Leprosy
- Trauma
- Abscess
- Syphilis

Parosmia:

- Perception of unpleasant smell in the absence of any disease process in the nose or sinuses
- Streptomycin toxicity, temporal lobe epilepsy

Some terms related to smell:

- Loss of sense of smell: Anosmia
- Perception of bad smell (maxillary sinusitis, foreign body in nose): Cacosmia

Atrophic rhinitis/ozaena:

- Caused by Klebsiella ozaenae (perez bacillus)
- Merciful anosmia
- Atrophied mucosa
- Roomy nasal cavity
- Management:
  - o Alkaline nasal douches
  - o Young's operation (closure of anterior nares)

Rhinoscleroma/Woody nose:

- Chronic granulomatous disease caused by Klebsiella rhinoscleromatosis (Frisch bacillus)
- Granulation tissue is made of plasma cells, Rusell bodies and Mikulicz cells
- Management: Streptomycin/Tetracycline

CSF rhinorrhoea:

- May be due to trauma or following endonasal surgery
- Leakage of watery, clear fluid from nose
- Patient cannot sniff it back
- No stiffening of handkerchief with the nasal discharge
- HRCT scan can identify a skull base defect associated with CSF rhinorrhea
- Management of non-surgical trauma:
  - o 8-10 days bed rest in head-up position
  - o Antibiotics
  - o Avoid coughing and sneezing

For better preparation and success in AIIMS-NORCET Exam, download **'drkamalkvgroup'** mobile app from Google Playstore.
WhatsApp: +91 84 7000 4333

SINUSITIS

Acute sinusitis:

- Order of involvement of sinuses: Maxillary > Frontal > Ethmoid > Sphenoid
- Caused by pneumococcus, H. influenzae

Maxillary sinusitis:

- Mucopurulent pus in middle meatus
- Maxillary tenderness
- Fever
- Bodyache

Frontal sinusitis:

- Periodicity (office headache: increases during mid-day and decreases by evening) and frontal tenderness
- Sinusitis absent at birth: Frontal sinusitis
- Common complication of frontal sinusitis: Pott's puffy tumour, mucocele

Sphenoid sinusitis:

- Postnasal drip
- Severe retro-orbital headache

Ethmoid sinusitis:

- Orbital cellulitis
- Most commonly seen in young children/infants

Management:

- Antibiotics
- Steam inhalation
- Analgesics

EPISTAXIS

Most common site:

- Keisselbach's plexus (area of anastomoses between ICA and ECA)
- In Little's area (Anteroinferior part of nasal septum)

Recurrent epistaxis is seen in:

- DNS/deviated nasal septum
- Atrophic rhinitis
- Maxillary Ca
- Angiofibroma (Most common cause of epistaxis in pubescent male)

Most common cause of epistaxis:

- In children: Trauma
- In adults: Hypertension

Management:

- Control BP if hypertensive
- Cold compress (causes reflex vasoconstriction)
- Nasal pinching for 5 minutes
- Anterior nasal packing (both sides)
- Cauterization with silver nitrate

III. THROAT

ORAL CAVITY

Ludwig's angina:

- Edema floor of mouth
- Involves submandibular
- Sublingual spaces

Ranula:

- Thin walled, retention cyst
- Sublingual

PHARYNX

Nasopharynx:

- Oval shaped
- Extends from base of skull to the level of soft palate/palatal sphincter (C2 vertebrae)
- Opening of eustachian tube
- Boundaries of nasopharynx:
  - o Roof: Basisphenoid, basiocciput
  - o Posterior wall: Anterior arch of atlas
- Pharyngeal opening of the eustachian tube:
  - o 1.25 cm behind the posterior end of inferior turbinate
  - o Located on the lateral wall
- Fossa of Rosenmuller/Pharyngeal recess:
  - o Located behind and above the eustachian tube opening
  - o Common site of Nasopharyngeal carcinoma

Oropharynx:

- From soft palate/palatal sphincter to the level of laryngeal inlet/tip of the epiglottis (C4)
- Boundaries:
  - o Anterior: Oral cavity
  - o Bottom: Laryngeal inlet
  - o Roof: Soft palate

Laryngopharynx/Hypopharynx:

- Extends from the upper margin of the epiglottis to the lower border of cricoid cartilage/upper end of esophagus (C6)

- 3 parts of hypopharynx/laryngopharynx:
  - o Posterior pharyngeal wall
  - o Post-cricoid region
  - o Pyriform sinus

Posterior pharyngeal wall:

- Extends from the upper margin of epiglottis to the upper end of the esophagus

Post-cricoid region:

- Lowest portion of hypopharynx
- Mucosa from upper to lower border of cricoid cartilage

Pyriform sinus:

- Recess on each side of larynx

TUMOURS OF PHARYNX

Juvenile nasopharyngeal angiofibroma:

- Affects young pubertal males
- Almost always seen in males
- Most common initial symptom is nasal obstruction
- Severe recurrent epistaxis is common Nature: Benign tumour common in South East Asia and India
- Vascular neoplasm (blood channels have no muscle coat, so may bleed more during surgery)
- Most common site: Posterior part of nasal cavity (close to spheno-palatine foramen)
- Tumour arising from a broad base in the roof of nasopharynx or lateral wall
- Investigation of choice: Contrast enhanced CT scan
- Treatment of choice: Surgery/A lateral rhinotomy (they are responsive to radiotherapy)

Nasopharyngeal carcinoma:

- Squamous cell carcinoma is the most common type
- Most common presentation: Neck mass/enlarged neck nodes
- Most common age group affected: Bimodal
- Most common site: Lateral wall of nasopharynx (Fossa of Rosenmuller/lateral pharnygeal recess)
- Associated with:
  - o EBV infection
  - o Cigarette smoking
  - o Consumption of salt cured fish which is high in nitrosamines
  - o Serous otitis media
- Modality for tumour mapping: CT scan
- Management: Radiotherapy

Peritonsillar abscess/quinsy:

- Severe throat pain, trismus, hot potato voice (altered voice quality)
- Unilateral bulging lateral and above the affected tonsil
- Tender cervical lymphadenopathy
- Torticollis
- Most common organism: Streptococcus
- Timing of surgery (quinsy tonsillectomy): 6 weeks after appearance
- Usually, bilateral tonsillectomy is done
- Tonsil with quinsy is easy to remove as abscess partially dissects the tonsil from the muscles of pharynx
- Aspiration and incision-drainage may be done

LARYNX

Anatomy:

- Extends from: Vertebrae C3 to C6
- Structure:
  - o Ligaments and muscles
  - o Cartilaginous framework
- Cartilages of larynx:
  - o Paired: Arytenoid
  - o Single:
    - – Thyroid
    - – Epiglottis
    - – Cricoid

Region of larynx:

- Supraglottis
- Glottis
- Subglottis

DISEASES OF THE LARYNX

Laryngomalacia:

- Most common cause of stridor in newborn
- Shape of epiglottis: Omega shaped epiglottitis
- Management: Reassurance (NO active treatment)

Vocal cord paralysis:

- Maximum stridor is seen with: Bilateral, Incomplete Vocal cord palsy
- Most dangerous vocal cord palsy: Bilateral, Abductor palsy
- Most common cause of vocal cord palsy: Total thyroidectomy
- Bilateral recurrent laryngeal nerve palsy occurs in:
  - o Thyroid malignancy
  - o Thyroidectomy

Acute epiglottitis:

- Most common in 2-7 years
- Most common causative organism for epiglottitis: H. influenzae type B
- Change in cry/voice is typical
- Dysphagia
- Thumb sign on X-ray
- Management: Antibiotics, tracheostomy for respiratory obstruction
- Most common cause of death in epiglottitis: Complete air-way obstruction
- There is marked swelling which may extend to the supraglottic tissues
- Inspiratory stridor

Croup/Laryngotracheobronchitis:

- Most common in 3 months to 3 years age group
- Bark of seal type of voice
- Stridor
- Low grade fever
- Steeple sign (Narrowing of subglottic region) is seen in: Croup (Most common caused by para influenza)
- Antibiotics

Laryngeal TB:

- Mamillated appearance
- Most common in posterior wall of larynx
- Turban epiglottis

MALIGNANT NEOPLASM OF LARYNX

Laryngeal carcinoma:

- Most common type is glottic carcinoma (60%)
- Most common in males
- Age >55 years
- Associated with smoking and alcohol
- Most common histological subtype: Squamous cell Ca
- Diagnosis can be made by:
  - o Flexible laryngoscope
  - o Biopsy or
  - o CT scan
- Management:
  - o Radiotherapy/RT for early stages
  - o RT + surgery for advanced stages

Supraglottic carcinoma:

- Most common manifestation: Pain is the most common manifestation
- Lymphatic spread: Early lymphatic spread to upper and middle jugular nodes
- May spread locally
- Nodal metastases occur early
- Bilateral metastases in epiglottic cancer
- Often silent
- Hoarseness is a late symptom
- Throat pain, dysphagia and referred pain in the ear or mass in lymph nodes in neck may be the presenting features

Glottic carcinoma:

- Earliest and most common manifestation: Hoarseness of voice because lesion of cord affects its vibratory capacity, so glottic cancers are detected early

- Prognosis: Best prognosis
- Lymphatic spread: No lymphadenopathy
- Most common type
- Free edge and upper surface of vocal cord in its anterior and middle third is the frequent site
- May spread locally and can involve other side as well
- Vocal cord mobility is unaffected in early stages
- Fixation of vocal cord indicates spread of disease to thyroarytenoid muscle and is a bad prognostic sign

TRACHEOSTOMY

High tracheostomy:

- Above the level of thyroid isthmus (above 2nd tracheal ring)
- NOT advocated as subglottic stenosis may occur

Mid tracheostomy:

- Preferred one
- Done through 2nd – 3rd tracheal rings

Low tracheostomy:

- Done below the level of isthmus of thyroid
- Tracheostomy tube may impinge on suprasternal notch

Tracheostomy tube:

- Double tube
- Made of titanium silver alloy

Structures damaged in emergency tracheostomy:

- Isthmus of thyroid
- Inferior thyroid vein
- Thyroid ima artery

Complications:

- One of the Common complications of tracheostomy: Tracheal stenosis (Mitomycin is used for this complication)

2 CHAPTER Obstetrical and Gynecological Nursing

SECTION 1: OBSTETRICS

I. ANATOMY AND PHYSIOLOGY

EMBRYOLOGY

Oogenesis:

- Oogonia (primitive germ cells) are derived from: Yolk sac
- Number at oogonia is maximum at 20th week: 7 million
- Oogonia enter prophase of the 1st meiotic division to become primary oocyte
- Total number of primary oocytes at birth: 2 million
- At puberty: 4 lakhs primary oocytes are left behind
- Out of this, some 400 are likely to ovulate during the entire reproductive period
- Primary oocyte has 22 pairs of autosomes (body characteristic) and 1 pair of sex chromosome (XX)
- Primary oocyte undergoes first meiotic division to form secondary oocyte (23, X) and one polar body (23, X)
- Ovulation occurs soon after the formation of secondary oocyte
- Secondary oocyte completes the second meiotic division only after fertilization, forming mature ovum and the second polar body
- In the absence of fertilization, the secondary oocyte does not complete the second meiotic division and degenerates

Fertilizable life span:

- Oocyte: 12-24 hours
- Sperm: 48-72 hours

Events after LMP:

- Secondary oocyte extrusion: day 14
- Secondary oocyte reaches tube
- Fertilization with extrusion of second polar body: Day 14-16
- Formation of zygote, 2-cell stage and 4-cell stage
- Early morula: Day 17
- Late morula: Day 18
- Early blastocyst stage with disappearance of zona pellucida: Day 19-20
- Early phase of implantation: Day 20-21

Fertilization:

- Most common site of fertilization: Ampulla
- Zygote reaches uterine cavity in which stage: 16 celled stage/ morula

Umbilical cord:

- Placental circulation is established on:
  - o Uteroplacental: 10-11th day
  - o Fetoplacental: 21-22nd day
- Vessels in umbilical cord: 2 arteries, 1 vein
- Nitabuch's layer (C): Zone of fibrinoid degeneration; where trophoblasts and decidua meet (in placenta)

Decidua:

- It is the endometrium of pregnancy
- D. basalis/serotina: In contact with base of blastocyst
- D. capsularis/reflexa: Covering the blastocyst
- D. vera/parietalis: Rest of the decidual lining outside the site of implantation

II. DIAGNOSIS OF PREGNANCY

AMNIOTIC FLUID

Features:

- Replaced every: 3 hours
- Alkaline with specific gravity of 1.010
- Amniotic fluid index/AFI:
  - o Abdomen is divided into 4 quadrants
  - o On USG, largest vertical pocket is measured in each quadrant
  - o Sum of the four measurements (in cms) is the AFI

Amount:

- At 12 weeks: 50 ml
- At 20 weeks: 400 ml
- Amount at term: 600-800 ml
- There is reduction in volume in the pregnancies continued post-term (200 ml at 43 weeks) maximum at: 36-38 weeks (1000 ml)

Amniotic fluid appearance:

- Normal: Pale straw colour (due to exfoliated lanugo and epidermal cells from fetal skin)
- Golden yellow: Rh incompatibility
- Green coloured (meconium stained) amniotic fluid indicates: Fetal distress in presentations other than breech/transverse (thick with presence of flakes suggest chronic fetal distress)
- Greenish yellow/saffron: Post-maturity
- Dark coloured: Concealed accidental hemorrhage
- Dark brown/tobacco juice: Intrauterine death

Abnormalities:

- Causes of oligohydramnios:
  - o Renal agenesis
  - o Multicystic dysplastic kidneys etc.
- Polyhydramnios is seen in:
  - o Esophageal atresia
  - o Duodenal atresia etc.

SIGNS OF PREGNANCY

Clinical signs and timings:

- Congestion of pelvis causing dusky/purplish hue of anterior vaginal wall and vestibule: Chadwick sign/Jacquemier's sign; 8 weeks
- Cyanosis and softening of cervix because of increased vascularity: Goodell's sign; 6 weeks
- Pregnant cervix feels like the lips of the mouth, while in the non-pregnant state, like that of tip of the nose
- Compressibility of isthmus on bimanual examination: Hegars sign; 6-10 weeks
  - o Upper part of the body of uterus is enlarged by growing fetus
  - o Lower part of the body is empty and extremely soft
  - o Cervix is comparatively firm
- One half of the uterus is more firm than the other half in lateral implantation: Piskaceks sign (asymmetrical enlargement of uterus in lateral implantation)
- Pulsations in lateral vaginal fornix: Osianders sign; 8 weeks
- Regular and rhythmic contractions of uterus, elicited by bimanual examination: Palmers sign;
  - o 4-8 weeks
  - o Valuable sign when elicited

ANTENATAL VISITS

Visits and timings:

- Minimum number of antenatal visit: 4

- o 1st around 16th week
- o 2nd between 24 and 28 weeks
- o 3rd at 32 weeks
- o 4th at 36 weeks
- Ideal number of antenatal visits: 12-14
  - o At an interval of 4 weeks up to 28 weeks (total of 7)
  - o At interval of 2 weeks up to 36 weeks (total of 4)
  - o Thereafter weekly till delivery

III. RELEVANT OSTEOLOGY

MATERNAL PELVIS

Types:

- Most common type: Gynaecoid (50%)
- Platypelloid/flat pelvis: Transverse diameter is more than AP diameter
- Least common type of pelvis: Platypelloid
- Deep transverse arrest/DTA and Persistent occipito posterior/POP position is common in: Android pelvis
- AP diameter more than transverse diameter: Anthropoid pelvis
- Face to pubis delivery is common in: Anthropoid pelvis

Diameters of pelvis:

- Shortest diameter of pelvic inlet:
  - o Obstetric conjugate (10 cm);
  - o Distance between the mid-point of the sacral promontory to prominent bony projection in the midline of the inner surface of the symphysis pubis
  - o It cannot be measured clinically but is inferred from diagonal conjugate by subtracting 3/4 inch (DC – 1.5 to 2 cm)

FETAL SKULL

Diameters:

- Shortest diameter of fetal skull:
  - o Bimastoid (7.5 cm)
  - o Distance between the tips of the mastoid processes
- Largest diameter of fetal skull:
  - o Mentovertical (14 cm)
  - o Extends from the mid-point of the chin to the highest point of sagittal suture

For better preparation and success in AIIMS-NORCET Exam, download **'drkamalkvgroup'** mobile app from Google Playstore.

WhatsApp: +91 84 7000 4333

IV. LABOR AND PUERPERIUM

BISHOP SCORING

Used for:

- Labor (It is a pre-induction cervical scoring system)

Includes:

- Dilatation of cervix
- Effacement of cervix
- Consistency of cervix
- Position of cervix
- Station of head
- Modification (1991) replaces effacement (%) with cervical length in cm

Score:

- Total score: 13
- Favorable score: 6-13
- Unfavorable score: 0-5

PARTOGRAM

Uses:

- Graphical representation of stages of labour
- Assessment of labour

Components:

- Fetal heart rate: Recorded every 30 minutes
- State of membranes: I (intact)
- Color of liquor: C (clear)/M (meconium stained)

- Cervical dilatation and descent of head
- Uterine contractions
- Drugs and fluids
- BP recorded every 2 hours
- Pulse recorded every 30 minutes

CERVICOGRAPH

Features:

- Graph showing relationship between cervical dilatation and labour
- Alert line: starts at 3 cm and ends at 10 cm dilatation (1 cm/hr)
- Action line: 3-4 hours to the right of alert line and parallel to it
- In a normal labor, the cervical dilatation should be either on the alert line or left to it

STAGES OF LABOR

1st stage:

- Onset of labor to dilatation of cervix
- 1st stage is concerned with preparation of the birth canal so as to facilitate expulsion of the fetus in second stage
- Average duration:
  - o About 12 hours in primigravidae
  - o 6 hours in multiparae
- 1st stage is clinically manifested by progressive uterine contraction, dilatation and effacement of cervix and ultimate rupture of membranes
- Main events in 1st stage:
  - o Dilatation and effacement of the cervix
  - o Full formation of lower uterine segment
- Phases:
  - o Latent phase (upto 3 cm of cervical dilatation)
  - o Active phase (upto 10 cm of cervical dilatation)

2nd stage:

- From full dilatation of cervix to complete birth of baby
- 2nd stage is concerned with the descent and delivery of the fetus through the birth canal
- Average duration:
  - o 2 hours in primigravidae
  - o 30 minutes in multiparae
- 2nd stage is clinically manifested by increased frequency and intensity of uterine contractions with appearance of "bearing down" efforts which result in expulsion of fetus
- Immediate care of newborn includes clearing the air passages and eyes, clamping and ligaturing of the umbilical cord and APGAR scoring
- Phases of 2nd stage:
  - o Propulsive: From full dilatation until head touches the pelvic floor
  - o Expulsive (bear down): Until the baby is delivered

3rd stage:

- Birth of infant to delivery of placenta
- 3rd stage comprises the phase of placental separation; its descent to the lower segment and finally its expulsion with the membranes
- Average duration of 3rd stage is 15 minutes
- The separation of placenta is achieved by marked reduction in the uterine surface area of the placental site following delivery due to retraction
- The placenta being inelastic shears off its attachment through the deep spongy decidual layer
- The bleeding is controlled by effective myomterial contraction and retraction (living ligature) and by thrombosis
- Oxytocin slow I/V or I/M or Methergin I/V is administered within one minute following the delivery of the baby

MECHANISM OF NORMAL LABOR

Features:

- Most common position is LOT/LOA
- Engaging anteroposterior diameter of the head is either suboccipito-bregmatic (9.5 cm) or suboccipito-frontal (10 cm)
- Engaging transverse diameter is biparietal (9.5 cm)

Principal movements:

- Engagement
- Descent
- Flexion
- Internal rotation
- Crowning
- Extension
- Restitution

- External rotation
- Expulsion of the trunk

Different steps:

- Engagement: When the greatest horizontal plane, the biparietal, has passed the plane of the pelvic brim, the head is said to be engaged
- Descent: It is because of uterine contraction and retraction, bearing down efforts and straightening of fetus
- Flexion: Full flexion of fetal head occurs as the head meets resistance of the birth canal during descent.
- Internal rotation:
  - o This is of great importance without which there will be no further descent
  - o Occiput comes to lie behind the symphysis pubis, rotating 1/8th of a circle
- Crowning:
  - o After internal rotation of the head, further descent occurs until the subocciput lies underneath the pubic arch
  - o At this stage, the maximum diameter of the head (biparietal diameter) stretches the vulval outlet without any recession of the head even after contraction is over – called "crowning of the head"
- Extension:
  - o Delivery of the head takes place by extension
  - o The successive parts of the fetal head to be born through the stretched vulval outlet are vertex, brow and face
- Restitution:
  - o It is the visible passive movement of the head due to untwisting of the neck sustained during internal rotation
  - o Movement of restitution occurs rotating the head through 1/8th of a circle in the direction opposite to that of internal rotation
  - o The occiput thus points to the maternal thigh of the corresponding side to which it originally lay
- External rotation:
  - o It is the movement of rotation of the head visible externally due to internal rotation of the shoulders
  - o As the anterior shoulder rotates towards the symphysis pubis from the oblique diameter, it carries the head in a movement of external rotation through 1/8th of a circle in the same direction as restitution
  - o The shoulders now lie in the anteroposterior plane
- Birth of shoulders and trunk:
  - o After the shoulders are positioned in anteroposterior diameter of the outlet, further descent takes place until the anterior shoulder escapes below the pubis symphysis first
  - o By the movement of lateral flexion of the spine, the posterior shoulder sweeps over perineum.
  - o The rest of the trunk is then expelled out by lateral flexion

LOCHIA

L. rubra:

- Reddish (1-4 days)
- Consists of blood, shreds of fetal membranes and decidua, vernix caseosa, lanugo and meconium

L. serosa:

- Yellowish (5-9 days)
- Consists of RBC but more leucocytes, wound exudates, mucus from the cervix and microorganisms (anaerobic streptococci and staphylococci)
- Presence of bacteria is not pathognomonic of infection

L. alba:

- Pale white (10-15 days)
- Contains plenty of decidual cells, leucocytes, mucus, cholestrin crystals, fatty and granular epithelial cells and microorganisms

Features:

- Duration: The normal duration may extend upto 3 weeks
- Clinical importance: Character of the lochial discharge gives useful information about the abnormal puerperal state

PUERPERIUM

Events:

- Puerperium lasts for:
  - o 6 weeks after delivery
  - o It is the period following childbirth during which the body tissues, specially the pelvic organs revert back approximately to the pre-pregnant state both anatomically and physiologically
- Uterus becomes a pelvic organ after:
  - o 2 weeks of delivery
  - o There is a steady decrease in uterine height by 1.25 cm (half inch)
- Involution of uterus is complete by:
  - o 6 weeks

- o Immediately following delivery, uterus weighs 1000 gm and measures 20 × 12 × 7.5 cm (length, breath and thickness)
- o At the end of 6 weeks, it weighs 60 gm and measures 8 × 5 × 1.25 cm

Puerperal sepsis:

- Most common cause of puerperal infection:
  - o Streptococcus haemolyticus group A (GAS)
  - o Streptococcus haemolyticus group B (GBS)
- Most common route of spread of puerperal infection:
  - o Direct spread
  - o Puerperal infection is essentially a wound infection
  - o Placental site (being a raw surface), lacerations of the genital tract (cervix, vagina, perineum) or caesarean section wounds may be infected

V. ABORTION

Definition of spontaenous abortion/miscarriage:

- Expulsion/extraction from its mother, of an embryo/fetus weighing 500 gm or less when it is not capable of independent survival
- This 500 gm of fetal development is attained approximately at 22 weeks (154 days) of gestation

1st trimester abortion:

- Causes: Genetic factors (50%), endocrine disorders (luteal phase defects/LPD, thyroid abnormalities, DM), immunological disorders (autoimmune), infection
- Most common cause of 1st trimester abortion: Autosomal trisomy (50%) (Most common is trisomy 16 amongst all trisomies – 30%)

Second trimester abortion:

- Management of cervical incompetence, which causes second trimester abortion: Circlage operation:
  - o Shirodkar's procedure
  - o McDonald's procedure
- Principle: The procedure reinforces the weak cervix by a non-absorbable tape, placed around the cervix at the level of internal OS
  - o Time of operation: Prophylactic cerclage should be done around 14 weeks of pregnancy or at least 2 weeks earlier than the lowest period of previous wastage, as early as 10th week

VI. ABNORMAL PREGNANCY

ECTOPIC PREGNANCY/EP

EP is associated with:

- Salpingitis/PID (Most common cause) increases the risk of ectopic pregnancy by 6-10 fold. Chlamydia trachomatis infection is the most common risk factor
- Tubal Endometriosis
- Progestasert IUD (highest rate of ectopic pregnancy)

Presentation:

- Pain (Most common)
- Classic triad of symptoms of disturbed tubal pregnancy are:
  - o Abdominal pain (100%)
  - o Preceded by amenorrhoea (75%)
  - o Lastly, appearance of vaginal bleeding (70%)
- Expelled products in EP have origin from: Decidua vera
- Most common type of EP which ruptures is:
  - o Tubal rupture is commoner in isthmic and interstitial implantation
  - o As the isthmic portion is narrow and the wall is less distensible, the wall may be easily eroded by chorionic villi
  - o Isthmic rupture usually occurs at 6-8 weeks and interstitial one at 4 months

Medical management of unruptured tubal EP:

- Salpingocentesis:
  - o Methotrexate
  - o Potassium chloride
  - o PGF2 alpha
  - o Hyperosmolar glucose
  - o Actinomycin-D etc.

- Requirements for starting medical management:
  - Serum HCG level <3000 IU/L
  - Tubal diameter <4 cm without any fetal cardiac activity
  - No intra-abdominal hemorrhage
- Monitoring is done by measuring beta-HCG on D4 and D7

HYDATID MOLE/VESICULAR MOLE

Pathology:

- Abnormal condition of the placenta where there are partly degenerative and partly proliferative changes in the young chorionic villi
- This results in formation of clusters of small cysts of varying sizes
- Because of its superficial resemblance to hydatid cyst, it is named as hydatidiform mole
- It is best regarded as benign neoplasia of the chorion with malignant potential

Symptoms:

- Most common presentation is vaginal bleeding (90%)
- Abdominal pain
- Expulsion of grape like vesicles per vaginum is diagnostic
- Molar pregnancy is usually diagnosed in:
  - 1st trimester
  - Patient gives a history of amenorrhoea of 8-12 weeks with initial features suggestive of normal pregnancy

Per abdomen:

- Size of uterus is more than the period of amenorrhoea (70%)
- Fetal parts not felt, nor any fetal movements
- Absence of fetal heart sounds

Per vaginal examination:

- Unilateral/bilateral enlargment of the ovary (theca lutein cyst)
- Finding of vesicles in the vaginal discharge is pathognomonic of H. mole

Complications:

- Haemorrhage and shock
- Sepsis
- Perforation of the uterus
- Pre-eclampsia
- Coagulation failure
- Choriocarcinoma (2-10%)

Treatment of choice:

- Suction – evacuation
  - It is safe, rapid and effective
  - Can be done even when the uterus is of 28 weeks gestation

Follow-up:

- Mandatory for all cases for at least 1 year, as occurrence of choriocarcinoma is confined to this period
- HCG levels following evacuation should regress to normal within 3 months time
- For 4-8 weeks, check up should be done once weekly
- After 56 days (when HCG is negative), for next 6 months, check up is done every one month

TWIN PREGNANCY

Types:

- Dizygotic/fraternal twins:
  - Most common (80%)
  - Results from fertilization of two ova
- Monozygotic/identical/uniovular:
  - 20%
  - Results from fertilization of a single ovum
- **Monozygotic twins**:
  - D/D (diamniotic – dichorionic)
  - 30%
  - Division takes place within 72 hours after fertilization (prior to morula stage)
  - Resulting embryos have 2 separate placenta, chorions and amnions
- D/M (Diamniotic - monochorionic):
  - 60%
  - Division takes place between the 4th to 8th day after formation of inner cell mass when chorion has already developed
- M/M (monoamniotic - monochorionic):
  - 3%
  - Division occurs after 8th day of fertilization, when the amniotic cavity has already formed

Conjoined twins:

- Most common type on conjoined twins: Thoracophagus
- Conjoined twins are extremely rare (1:100,000 to 1:50,000)

Perinatal mortality in twins:

- Most common cause: Prematurity
- 4-5 times higher than a singleton pregnancy
- Extremely high in monoamniotic monozygotic twins due to cord entanglement

COMPLICATED PREGNANCY

Types of Breech:

- Complete/flexed breech
- Frank/extended breech
- Footling breech

Footling breech:

- Engagement is late
- Elective caesarean section is indicated
- Worst prognosis
- Maximum chances of cord compression

Frank/extended breech:

- Hip is flexed
- Knee extended
- Engagement occurs earliest
- Seen in primigravidae
- External cephalic version is unsuccessful
- Least chances of cord compression

Complete/flexed breech:

- Knees and hip flexed
- Most common type
- External cephalic version is successful
- Seen in multipara
- Intermediate chances of cord compression

Shoulder dystocia:

- Predisposing factors:
  - o Anencephaly
  - o Fetal ascites
  - o Fetal macrosomia
  - o Obesity
  - o Diabetes postmaturity
  - o Associated with prolonged labor
- Fetal Complications:
  - o Brachial plexus injury
  - o Fracture of clavicle/humerus
- Maternal complications:
  - o Uterine rupture
  - o Perineal tears
  - o Hemorrhage
- Management steps:
  - o Apply suprapubic pressure (never apply fundal pressure as it causes further impaction of the shoulder and may cause orthopedic/neurological damage)
  - o McRobert's manoeuvre
  - o Wood's corckscrew manoeuvre
  - o Extraction of posterior arm
  - o Cleidotomy

VII. MEDICAL DISORDERS IN PREGNANCY

Rh INCOMAPTIBILITY

Pathology:

- Also known as Immune hydrops/IH
- Alloimmunization/isoimmunization is defined as production of immune antibodies in an individual in response to foreign red cell antigen derived from another individual of the same species provided, the first one lacks antigen
- Mother is Rh –ve (D -ve)
- Fetus/husband is Rh +ve
- In alloimmunization, it is the IgG antibodies that cross the placenta and damage the fetus
- Degree of affection of fetus depends upon the degree of destruction of the fetal RBC by the antibodies
- Alloimmunization is preventable by the anti-D Ig prophylaxis
- It should be given within 72 hours of delivery

Indications of anti-D immunoprophylaxis in Rh (D) negative women are:

- Miscarriage

- Ectopic pregnancy
- MTP
- Chorionic villous sampling
- Amniocentesis
- One dose of anti-D (300 mcg) Ig is given prophylactically at around 28 weeks and a second dose is given after delivery within 72 hours if the infant is Rh (D) positive

Management is:

- Immediate cord ligation (to minimize even minute amount of antibody to cross to the fetus from the mother)
- The cord should be kept long (15-20 cm) for exchange transfusion, if required
- Anti-D Ig (I/M) to mother (with 72 hours)
- To prevent active immunization of Rh -ve yet unimmunized, Rh anti-D Ig is administered I/M to the mother following child birth
- It should be given provided the baby born is Rh +ve and direct Coomb's test is -ve

Dose of anti-D Ig:

- Following delivery: 300 mcg
- Induced/spontaneous abortion, ectopic/molar pregnancy or CVS in first trimester: 50 mcg
- Women with pregnancy >12 weeks: 300 mcg (full dose)

HEART DISEASES/HD AND PREGNANCY

Most common HD associated with pregnancy:

- Mitral stenosis/MS
- Symptoms of MS appears when the stenosis narrows mitral valve area to less than 2.5 cm^2
- In symptomatic cases, mortality ranges between 5 -15%
- Best time of surgery: 14-18 weeks

Conditions in which pregnancy is to be terminated:

- Primary pulmonary HTN
- Eisenmenger syndrome etc.

Risk of maternal mortality (%) with heart diseases:

- Minimal risk (ASD, VSD, PDA, corrected TOF): 0-1%
- Moderate risk (MS, AS, uncorrected TOF): 5-15%
- Major risk (Pulmonary HTN, COA): 25-50%

HIV AND PREGNANCY

HIV and AIDS:

- HIV is an incurbale infection that finally leads to terminal disease called AIDS
- 25-30% are women
- 90% of them are 20-49 years of age

Virus:

- HIV viruses (HIV-1 and HIV-2) are RNA retroviruses having the enzyme reverse transcriptase, which permits genomic RNA to be transcribed into double stranded DNA
- Virus attaches to T lymphocytes known as CD_4^+ cells (which combat viruses and bacteria)
- There is gradual depletion of CD_4^+ cells
- This leads to progressive loss of host immune defense and development of AIDS
- CD_4^+ count <200 cells/mm^3 is diagnostic of AIDS
- Median time from infection to AIDS is about 10 years

Perinatal transmission:

- Vertical transmission: 14-25%
  - o HIV-1: 15-40%
  - o HIV-2: 1-4%
- Risk is directly proportional to maternal viral load (HIV-RNA) and inversely to maternal immune status (CD_4^+count)

Diagnosis:

- Screening: ELISA (sensitivity 99.5%)
- PCR can be done
- Confirmatory: Western blot test/Immunofluorescence assay (IFA)
- Western blot detects specific viral antigens (p24/capsid, GP41/envelope and GP120/160)
- False positive WB test: <1 in 10,000

Incidence of perinatal transmission of HIV can be reduced by:

- Antiretroviral prophylaxis:
  - o HAART (Highly active antiretroviral therapy) to HIV-1 positive women reduces viral load (HIV RNA)
  - o Triple chemotherapy is preferred (2 drugs from NRTI + 1 from NNRTI/PI)
  - o Started between 14-28 weeks
  - o In resource poor settings: Zidovudine reduces perinatal transmission from 25% to 7%
- LSCS at 38 weeks for women taking HAART:
  - o Who have plasma viral load >50 copies/mL
  - o Elective CS reduces the risk of vertical transmission by 50%
- Intrapartum nevirapine:

- o A single dose of Nevirapine at the onset of labor and a single dose of it to the newborn at age 48 hours is an effective alternative requirement for women who had no prior therapy
- Avoid breastfeeding:
  - o Breastfeeding double the risk of MTCT (from 14 to 28%) but where alternative forms of nutrition are not safe, the risk associated with breastfeeding may be accepted.

PREGNANCY INDUCED HYPERTENSION/PIH

PIH includes:

- Gestational hypertension (BP 140/90 mm Hg for the first time in pregnancy after 20 weeks, without proteinuria)
- Pre-eclampsia (Gestational HTN with proteinuria)
- Eclampsia (Pre-eclampsia complicated with convulsions and/or coma)

Pathological organ changes:

- Blood: Thrombocytopenia, coagulopathy
- Uteroplacental bed: Placental abruption, IUGR
- Kidney: Proteinuria, oliguria
- Liver: Necrosis, raised level of AST and ALT
- CNS: Seizures, posterior reversible encephalopathy, cortical blindness

Management objectives:

- Control BP
- Prevent complications like eclampsia
- Termination of the pregnancy is the only definitive treatment of pre-eclampsia

Pre-eclampsia:

- Syndrome of multiple organ dysfunction
- Manifest first time beyond the 20th week
- Characterised by the appearance of hypertension to the extent of 140/90 mm Hg or more and proteinuria with or without pathological edema
- Basic pathology is endothelial dysfunction and vasospasm

Earliest sign of pre-eclampsia:

- Raised BP
- DBP usually tends to rise first followed by the SBP

Symptom of pre-eclampsia:

- Rapid gain in weight (earliest)
  - o A rapid gain in weight of more than 5 lb a month or more than 1 lb a week in later months of pregnancy is significant
- Blurring, scotomata, dimness of vision or at time complete blindness in PIH is due to: Retinal infarction, Retinal detachment
  - o Vision is usually regained within 4-6 weeks following delivery
  - o Reattachment of the retina occurs following subsidence of oedema and normalization of BP after delivery
- Complications of pre-eclampsia:
  - o Eclampsia
  - o HELLP syndrome
  - o Accidental hemorrhage
  - o Dimness of vision/blindness
  - o Cerebral hemorrhage
  - o ARDS

Treatment:

- DOC in severe pre-eclampsia (a persistent rise of SBP >160 mm Hg or DBP >110 mm Hg, protein excretion >5 gm/day, Oliguria <400 ml/day, platelet count <1 lakh/mm^3, HELLP syndrome, cerebral/visual disturbances): Methyldopa (central and peripheral anti-adrenergic action)

Eclampsia:

- Eclampsia is defined as: HTN, proteinuria, edema and convulsions
- Pre-eclampsia when complicated by generalised tonic-clonic convulsions and/or coma is called eclampsia
- Most common eclampsia is: Ante partum type (50%)

Treatment for controlling convulsions in eclampsia:

- Magnesium sulphate
- Ideally the patient should be delivered within a period of 6-8 hours even if the fits are controlled
- It acts as a membrane stabilizer and neuroprotector
- It has got no detrimental effects on the neonate within therapeutic levels
- It does not control hypertension

Toxicity of $MgSO_4$ is monitored by:

- Knee jerk
- Respiratory rate
- Urinary output
- Therapeutic level of $MgSO_4$: 4-7 mEq/L

- Repeat injections are given only if the knee jerks are present, urine output is > 30 ml/hour and the respiration rate is >12 per minute

VIII. COMPLICATIONS OF LABOR

Complications of 3rd stage of labor:

- Postpartum hemorrhage (Most common)
- Retention of placenta
- Shock – hemorrhagic and non-hemorrhagic
- Pulmonary embolism (amniotic fluid/air)
- Uterine inversion (rare)

POSTPARTUM HEMORRHAGE

Most common cause of PPH:

- Atonic uterus (80%)
- With the separation of the placenta, the uterine sinuses are torn, cannot be compressed effectively due to imperfect contraction and retraction of the uterine musculature and bleeding continues

PPH is said to occur if:

- Blood loss is more than 500 cc
- The average blood loss following vaginal delivery, caesarean delivery and caesarean hysterectomy is 500 ml, 1000 ml and 1500 ml respectively

Drugs used for PPH:

- Misoprostol (PGE_1)
- Ergometrine
- Oxytocin

Management of atonic uterus causing PPH:

- Step I:
  - o Massage the uterus to make it hard
  - o I/V oxytocin infusion
  - o Inj. Methergin I/V
  - o Examine expelled placenta
- Step II: Explore uterus under GA
- Step III: Uterine massage and bimanual compression
- Step IV: Tight intrauterine packing under GA
- Step V: Surgical method to control PPH (Ligation of arteries, B-lynch compression suture, arterial embolization or hysterectomy)

UTERINE INVERSION

Cause of uterine inversion (uterus is turned inside out partially or completely):

- Mismanaged 3rd stage of labor/faulty technique in manual removal (pulling the cord when the uterus is atonic specially combined with fundal pressure) Spontaneous (40%)

IX. DIAGNOSTIC OBSTETRICS

CHORIONIC VILLOUS SAMPLING/CVS

CVS:

- Prenatal diagnosis of genetic disorders
- Material for study: Trophoblast cells
- Fetal loss: 0.5-1%
- Accurate; may need amniocentesis
- MTP is safe (1st trimester), if needed as per report
- A few villi are collected from the chorion frondosum under USG
- Anti-D (50 mcg IM) should be administered to Rh negative woman
- CVS is preferably done at:
  - o 10-12 weeks (transcervically)
  - o Trans-abdominally: 10 weeks to term

HCG

HCG:

- Rescue and maintenance of corpus luteum till 6 weeks of pregnancy

- HCG is secreted by: Synctiotrophoblasts (principal site of protein and steroid hormones in pregnancy)
- Structurally HCG has:
  - o Glycoprotein with molecular weight of 36000-40000
  - o 2 subunits (alpha and beta)
  - o Alpha subunit is biochemical similar to LH
  - o Beta subunit is relatively unique to HCG
- Act as a stimulus for secretion of progesterone by the corpus luteum of pregnancy
- Plasma half life: 36 hours
- Can be detected in maternal serum as early as 8-9 days post fertilization
- Doubling time: 1.4-2 days
- Maximum blood and urine levels: 100-200 ID between 60 and 70 days
- Disappears from circulation within 2 weeks following delivery

High HCG levels:

- Multiple pregnancies
- H. mole/choriocarcinoma
- Down syndrome

Low HCG levels:

- Ectopic pregnancies
- Spontaneous abortion

FETAL HEART RATE/FHR

Early deceleration (Type I dips)

- Head compression (vagal nerve activation)
- Type I dips are uniform, repetitive periodic slowing of FHR
- Onset, nadir and recovery of deceleration coincides with the beginning, peak and ending of uterine contractions

Late deceleration (Type II dips):

- Uteroplacental insufficiency and fetal hypoxia (5%)
- Type II dips are uniform, repetitive periodic slowing of FHR with onset mid toe end of uterine contraction and nadir >20 seconds after the peak of the contraction and FHR retrun to normal after the contraction is over

BIOPHYSICAL PROFILE/BPP

BPP predicts:

- +/- of fetal asphyxia

5 Parameters in BPP:

- NST (Non-stress test)
- Fetal breathing
- Gross body movements of fetus
- Fetal muscle tone
- Amniotic fluid

X. DRUGS IN OBSTETRICS

Indicated in pregnancy:

- Anti-thyroid: Propylthiouracil
- Anti-TB: INH
- Anti-coagulant: Heparin
- Anti-TB: INH
- Anti-malarial: Chloroquine

Contraindicated in pregnancy:

- All live vaccines
- Yellow fever vaccine, being a live vaccine can be given in special circumstances
- Anti-TB: Streptomycin
- Anti-malarial: Primaquine
- Anti-convulsant: Valproate (causes NTD)
- Anti-folate: Methotrexate
- Anti-hypertensives: ACE inhibitors

For better preparation and success in AIIMS-NORCET Exam, download **'drkamalkvgroup'** mobile app from Google Playstore.

WhatsApp: +91 84 7000 4333

SECTION 2: GYNECOLOGY

I. RELEVANT ANATOMY AND PHYSIOLOGY

PELVIC ORGANS AND STRUCTURES

Fallopian tube:

- Situated in the medial 3/4th of the upper free margin of the broad ligaments
- 2 openings: Uterine (1 mm in diameter) and pelvic/abdominal ostium (2 mm in diameter)
- 4 parts:
  - o Intramural/interstitial: ½ inch in length (L) and 1 mm in diameter (D)
  - o Isthmus: 1 inch (L) and 2.5 mm (D)
  - o Ampulla: 2 inch (L)
  - o Infundibulum: ½ inch (L) and 6 mm (D)
- Blood supply:
  - o Uterine and ovarian artery
  - o Venous drainage through pampiniform plexus into ovarian veins
- Lined by: Ciliated columnar epithelium
- Length: 10 cms

Female urethra:

- Length: 4 cm (diameter: 6 mm)
- Lining: Transitional epithelium (except at the external urethral meatus where it becomes stratified squamous)

Uterus:

- Measures 8 cm and weighs 50-80 grams
- Isthmus is bounded above by the anatomical internal os and below by the histological internal os

Ovary:

- Attached to posterior leaf of the broad ligament by the mesovarium
- Ovarian fossa is related posteriorly to the ureter

PHYSIOLOGY

Ovulation:

- Best predictor of ovulation: Pre-ovulatory rise in LH
- Sustained peak level of estradiol for about 24 hours beyond 200 pg/mL in late follicular phase results in LH surge (positive feedback effect)
- Ovulation occurs approximately 32-36 hours after the onset of LH surge and about 10-12 hours after the LH peak
- The mean duration of LH surge is about 24 hours
- After ovulation, the ruptured Graafian follicle becomes corpus luteum
- Regression of CL starts on day 22-23 of infertile cycle
- LH hormone, with adequate number of LH receptors in the granulosa cells (as induced during folliculogenesis) with increased secretion of estradiol, is the key factor of adequate corpus luteum formation
- Ovulatory period: Corresponds to 14 days before next menstruation
- LH stimulates: Follicle rupture and ovulation
- Primary oocyte undergoes first meiotic division giving rise to secondary oocyte and one polar body just prior to ovulation
- The secondary oocyte completes the second meiotic division only after fertilization by a sperm in the fallopian tube
- One follicle with highest antral concentration of estrogen and lowest androgen : estrogen ratio and the granulosa cells containing the maximum receptors for FSH becomes the dominant follicle
- Both FSH and LH regulates the follicular development
- LH surge is followed by ovulation
- After ovulation, the ruptured graafian follicle becomes corpus luteum

Corpus luteum:

- In normal menstrual cycle, progesterone is secreted by: Corpus luteum
- Corpus luteum secretes estrogen and progesterone both

Menstruation:

- Amount of blood loss in menstruation: Up to 80 ml (average 35 mL)
- Average age of menarche: 13 years
- Average loss of iron in each menses: 13 mg

II. GYNECOLOGICAL INFECTIONS

Senile/atrophic vaginitis:

- Vaginitis in post-menopausal women
- Atrophy of vulvovaginal structures due to estrogen deficiency
- Vaginal defense is lost
- Managed by systemic estrogen/local estrogen cream application

Trichomonas vaginitis:

- Most common (STD) cause of vaginitis in childbearing age
- Sudden profuse and offensive vaginal discharge
- Irritation and itching
- Urinary symptoms (dysuria and frequency)
- Thin, greenish-yellow and frothy offensive discharge per vaginum
- Vulva is inflammed with evidence of pruritis
- Vaginal walls become red and inflammed with multiple punctate hemorrhagic spots
- Managed by metronidazole
- Husband should be given the same treatment schedule
- Until the wife is cured, husband should use barrier contraceptive

Candida vaginitis/Moniliasis:

- Candida albicans is a gram-positive yeast-like fungus
- Predisposing conditions: Diabetes, pregnancy, antibiotics, HIV
- Vaginal discharge with intense vulvovaginal pruritis
- Pruritis is out of proportion to the discharge
- Discharge is thick, curdy white and in flakes (cottage cheese type) often adherent
- Removal of white flakes reveals multiple oozing spots
- Correction of predisposing conditions
- Local fungicidal preparations (cream/pessary) are used (nystatin, clotrimazole, miconazole)
- Single dose oral therapy with fluconazole/itraconazole
- Treat the partner simultaneously

Bacterial vaginosis:

- Caused by Gardnerella/haemophilus vaginalis and anaerobic organisms (Bacteroides species, Peptococcus species, mobiluncus and Mycoplasma hominis)
- Marked reduction in lactobacilli
- Creamy (homogenous, greyish-white) and adherent vaginal discharge with fishy smell without evidence of inflammation
- Managed with oral metronidazole
- Clindamycin cream and metronidazole gel are recommended for vaginal application
- Treat the partner simultaneously

Gonorrhoea:

- Caused by N. gonorrhoae: Gram negative diplococcus
- Principal sites of involvement are endocervix, urethra, Skene's gland and Bartholin's gland (columnar and transitional epithelium)
- Squamous epithelium is resistant to gonococcal invasion, so vaginitis in adults is not possible
- 50% cases are asymptomatic
- Urinary symptoms (dysuria)
- Irritant vaginal mucopurulent discharge
- On squeezing the urethra and giving pressure on the Bartholin's glands, purulent exudate escapes
- Managed by single dose regimen of ceftriaxone/ciprofloxacin/ofloxacin/cefixime/levofloxacin
- Culture should be made 7 days after therapy
- Repeat culture should be made at monthly intervals following menses for three months
- If the reports are persistently negative, the patient is declared cured

Lymphgranuloma venerum/LGV:

- Caused by L serotypes of Chlamydia trachomatis
- Initial lesion is painless papule, pustule or ulcer in the vulva, urethra, rectum or the cervix
- Inguinal nodes are involved (feels rubbery)
- Acute lymphangitis and lymphadenitis

- Lymphatic obstruction leads to vulval elpehantiasis
- Glands become necrosed and abscess (bubo) forms
- Bubo ruptures and multiple draining sinuses and fistula forms
- Classical clinical sign is groove sign
- Manage with Doxycycline/azithromycin/erythromycin
- Treat the partner as well

Chancroid/Soft sore:

- Caused by: H. ducreyi (Gram-negative streptobacillus)
- Presents as: Genital ulcer (painful)
- Lesion start as multiple vesiculopustules over the vulva, vagina or cervix
- It then sloughs to form shallow ulcers
- Lesion is very tender (there may be cluster of ulcers)
- Inguinal adenitis (inguinal buboes)
- Unilateral inguinal lymphadenitis may occur which may suppurate to form abscess (buboes)
- DOC: Azithromycin/Ceftriaxone/Ciprofloxacin/Co-trimoxazole

Syphilis:

- Caused by Treponema pallidum
- Hard chancre of primary syphilis is painless with an indurated base
- VDRL and TPHA tests are used for screening and FTA-abs is used for confirmation
- I/M Benzathine penicillin is used for treatment

Quick Recap:

- Profuse curdy, white discharge (cottage cheese appearance), intense itching: Candidiasis
- Trichominiasis:
  - o Caused by: Trichomonas vaginalis (flagellate parasite)
  - o Clinical presentation: Profuse, thin, frothy, greeny discharge (malodorous)
  - o Appearance of vagina: Strawberry vagina
  - o DOC: Metronidazole
- Bacterial vaginosis:
  - o Caused by: Multibacterial
    - – Hemophilus vaginalis
    - – Gardnerella
    - – Mobiluncus (corkscrew spinning anaerobe)
  - o Clinical presentation: White, Milky, homogenous and adherent discharge
  - o Vaginal pH: Alkaline (greater than 4.5)
  - o Histological feature: Clue cells
  - o DOC: Metronidazole

GENITAL TB

- Most common site of primary TB infection in body:
  - o Lungs (50%)
  - o Lymph nodes (40%)
- Most common site of affection in genital TB: Fallopian tubes
- Pelvic organs are affected secondarily, the primary site is predominantly in lung
- Spread is by hematogenous route
- Fallopian tubes are almost always affected (100%) bilaterally
- Infertility present in 70% of cases
- Menorrhagia may be the early symptom but more commonly, the patient presents with oligomenrrhoea/amenorrhoea
- Treatment:
  - o 4 drugs ATT (RIPE) Initial phase for 2 months
  - o 2 drugs ATT (RI) Continuation phase for 4 months
- In terms of future reproduction, prognosis is most unfavourable
- Pregnancy rate is rare (5-10%)
- Ectopic pregnancy is more (40%)
- Pregnancy rarely goes up to full term

III. CONTRACEPTION

Barrier methods:

- Ideal contraceptive for couple staying away and meeting occasionally: Barrier contraception
- Barrier methods (both male and female), apart from their contraceptive effect, have the advantages of preventing transmission of sexually transmitted diseases, HIV and reducing the incidence of cancer cervix by preventing viral transmission

OCPs:

- Ideal contraceptive for newly married couple: OCP

- OCP of choice in lactating females is:
  - o Minipill/progesterone only pill/POP
  - o POP are safe in a lactating woman and can be started six weeks onwards
  - o POPs are particularly useful when estrogen is contraindicated or its side effects are intolerable
  - o POP is as effective as IUCD, but less effective than COP
- OCP protects against:
  - o Endometriosis (Causes non-ovulation)
  - o Uterine Ca
  - o Ovarian Ca
  - o The incidence of Ovarian Ca is reduced by 40% and uterine malignancy by 50% if taken for one year, and this effect lasts as long as 10 years after stoppage
  - o Reduces menstrual loss (so prevents anemia and is useful in menorrhagia and polymenorrhoea)

IUCD:

- IUCD is an established method of female contraception in India on account of one time insert
- Progesterone impregnated IUCD has an added advantage of reducing menstrual bleeding, but is expensive

Emergency contraception/EC/post-coital contraception:

- It is a technique to prevent conception if rape/unprotected intercourse occur around ovulation
- Yields 95-98% success and avoids MTP
- LNG/Levonorgestrel tablet:
  - o It contains 0.75 mg LNG
  - o One tablet taken within 72 hours of intercourse and another 12 hours later is 98.9% successful
  - o The tablets can be taken upto 120 hours, but efficacy decreases with the longer coital drug interval
- RU 486 (Mifepristone) 10 mg single dose is effective in 99.1%
- Others include prostaglandin and insertion of Copper T

IV. GYNECOLOGICAL MALIGNANCIES

CERVICAL CA

Pathology:

- Arises from: Squamocolumnar junction
- Most common agent: HPV 16
- Other type of HPV which are associated with cervical Ca: HPV 18, 31, 45, 51, 52 and 53
- Other risk factors:
  - o Early sexual intercourse
  - o Multiple sexual partners

Features:

- Earliest symptom: Post-coital bleeding
- Other features: pelvic pain, cervical discharge

Prognosis:

- 100% cure rates are seen in: CIS (carcinoma-in-situ)
- Most common cause of death: Renal failure

FIBROID

Pathology:

- Most common type of fibroid: Intramural/interstitial (75%)
- Most fibroid starts as: Intramural/interstitial fibroids
- Most common to undergo malignant change (0.5%, rare before the age of 40):
  - o Intramural
  - o Submucous
- Most common type of degeneration: Hyaline (starts from the centre)

ENDOMETRIAL CARCINOMA

Predisposing factors:

- Family history
- Obesity
- DM
- Tamoxifen therapy
- PCOD

Treatment of atypical endometrial hyperplasia:

- Hysterecetomy (panhysterectomy in elderly)

V. MENSTRUAL DISORDERS

ENDOMETRIOSIS

Pathology:

- Presence of ectopic endometrial tissue outside the true cavity of the uterus
- Endometriosis manifests as islands of flame-shaped chocolate deposits or appear like powder burn marks
- Patient presents with pelvic pain, dyspareunia, menstrual disturbances and infertility
- Medical treatment consists of analgesics to control pain.
- Cyclic hormonal therapy and GnRH analogues provide relief from pain and help regress

MENOPAUSE

Premature menopause:

- When menstruation ceases before 40 years of age. Delayed menopause is one when the menopause fails to occur even beyond 55 years

Menopause:

- Permanent cessation of menstruation at the end of reproductive life due to ovarian follicular inactivity
- Average age being 50 years
- Genetically predetermined
- Gradual levels of first the FSH and then LH
- Estradiol levels falls to the optimal 20 pg/ml when menopause sets in
- Increased androgen secretion from the ovarian stroma and from adrenal
- Diagnosis is by classical symptom of 'hot flush' (50%) and confirmed elevated FSH levels to >100 mIU/ml and serum estradiol level <20 pg/ml

AMENORRHOEA

Physiology and pathology:

- Physiological before puberty, during pregnancy and lactation and following menopause
- Most common cause of amenorrhoea in a woman of reproductive age is pregnancy
- Regular menstruation indicates cyclical ovarian function in response to intact Hypothalamo-Pituitary-Ovarian/HPO axis
- Amenorrhoea/oligomenrrhoea indicates ovarian, endometrial and/or HPO axis dysfunction

Primary amenorrhea:

- Failure of menses in a girl by 16 years of age (regardless of the presence of secondary sexual characters)
- Failure of menses in a girl by 14 years of age (in the absence of secondary sexual characters)

Secondary amenorrhoea:

- Most common pathological cause of secondary amenorrhea (absence of menstruation for 6 months or more in a woman in whom normal menstruation has been established)
    - o In India: Endometrial TB
    - o Worldwide: Hypothalamic dysfunction

VI. GENITAL PROLAPSE

Pathology:

- Prolapse of pelvic organs into vaginal wall
- Important risk factors for prolapse is history of vaginal birth and the age of the woman

Degree of uterine prolapse:

- 1st: Uterus descends but external os remains in the vagina
- 2nd: External os protrudes outside the vagina but uterine body remains inside
- 3rd: Uterine body descends outside the vaginal introitus (procidentia)

VII. DRUGS USED IN GYNECOLOGY

Clomiphene:

- Used in the treatment of:
  - o PCOS (Stein Levinthal syndrome)
  - o In vitro fertilization
  - o Anovulatory fertility

Tamoxifen:

- Antiestrogenic (Non steroidal)
- Acts by binding to and reducing the availability of estrogen receptors

Danazol:

- Used in:
  - o Endometriosis
  - o Cyclic and non-cyclic mastalgia
  - o Primary menorrhagia
  - o Precocious puberty

For better preparation and success in AIIMS-NORCET Exam, download **'drkamalkvgroup'** mobile app from Google Playstore.

WhatsApp: +91 84 7000 4333

3 CHAPTER Pediatrics & Child Health Nursing

I. GROWTH AND DEVELOPMENT

Important milestones:

- Child smiles at familiar persons (social smile): 2 months
- Head control (neck holding): 3 months
- Sits with own support (tripod fashion): 6 months
- Sits without support: 8 months
- Says mama dada: 10 months
- Crawls: 11 months
- Copies circle: 3 years
- Knows age and sex: 3 years
- Can draw a rectangle: 4 years
- Can draw a triangle: 5 years

Important development milestones:

- 1 month: Turns head toward sound
- 2 months: Social smile
- 3 months: Neck holding, recognize mother
- 4 months: Grasp a rattle/ring when placed in hand
- 5 months: Bidextrous grasp (hold objects with both hands)
- 6 months: Roll over, monosyllables (ma; ba), smiles at mirror image
- 7 months: Palmar grasp
- 8 months: Plays 'peek a boo'
- 9 months: Standing with support, pincer grasp, bisyllables (mama, baba)
- 10-11 months: Walking with support
- 12 months: Standing alone without support, says two words with meaning
- 13 months: Walking without support
- 18 months: Can feed himself with slight spilling, says 10 words with meaning
- 24 months: Walking upstairs, draws horizontal/vertical line, says simple sentence
- 36 months: Waking upstairs with alternate steps, can dress/undress, tells a story

Neonate:

- Perinatal period: 28 weeks gestation to 7 days post-natal age
- Early neonatal period: First 7 days of life
- Late neonatal period: 8-28 days after birth

Body parameters

- Body weight doubles at: 5 months
- Body weight triples at: 1 year
- Body length increases in 1st year by: 25 cm (50% of birth length)

Growth in children:

- Weight at birth: 3 Kg
- Length at birth: 50 cm
- Head circumference at birth: 33-35 cm

Weight gain:

- Up to 3 months: 200 grams/week

- 3-6 months: 150 grams/week
- 6-12 months: 100 grams/week
- 1-6 years (preschool): 2 Kg/year
- >6 years (school going): 3 Kg/year

Increase in length/height:

- 1st year: 25 cm
- 2nd year: 12.5 cm
- 3 years till puberty: 6 cm/year
- >2 years, height can be calculated as: Age (years) + 77 cm

II. NUTRITIONAL DISORDERS

Protein Energy Malnutrition:

- Indicators are:
  - o Weight
  - o Height
  - o Mid arm circumference/MAC (<12.5 indicates severe malnutrition)
  - o Quetlet index
  - o Dugdale index etc.
- Age independent indicators:
  - o Bangle test
  - o Shakir tape
  - o MAC
  - o Kanawati index (MAC/head cricumference)
  - o QUAC stick
- Earliest indicator of PEM is low weight for age (includes both acute and chronic malnutrition)

Nutritional dwarfism:

- Normal birth weight with subsequent retardation (Weight/Age and Height/Age are low but Weight/Height may be normal)
- Delayed bone age

Kwashiorkor:

- Altered mentation (apathic)
- Flag sign
- Hepatomegaly (fatty liver)
- Poor appetite
- Dermatosis (flaky paint, crazy pavement)

Marasmus:

- Wasting (old man appearance)
- Weight <60%
- Alert
- Good appetite

Quick recap:

- Edema is seen in: Kwashiorkar
- Hepatomegaly is seen in: Kwashiorkar
- Acute malnutrition is judged by: Weight for height (Low W/H is wasting; <80%)
- Chronic malnutrition is judged by: Height for age (Low H/A is stunting; <90%; signifies duration of malnutrition)
- Wasting and stunting both signifies acute on chronic malnutrition
- Flag sign is seen in: Kwashiorkor

Rickets:

- Softened calvariae is known as: Craniotabes
- Prominent costochondral junction: Rachitic rosary
- Pot belly is because of : Hypotonia
- Bowing of legs: Genu varum
- Biochemical values:
  - o Low serum calcium and phosphate
  - o Raised alkaline phosphatase and PTH
- X-ray:
  - o Widening of metaphysic
  - o Cupping and splaying of metaphysis

Scurvy:

- Bleeding into skin and joints
- Pseudoparalysis
- X-ray:
  - o Wimburger sign
  - o White line of Frenkel
  - o Pelkan spur etc.

III. CONGENITAL DISORDERS

Down syndrome:

- Most common trisomy is: Down syndrome
- Brachycephalic skull
- Hypotonia
- Palpebral fissure slopes upwards
- Marked epicanthic folds
- Brushfield's spots
- Increased nuchal fold thickness
- Simian crease (single palmar crease)
- Most common associated cardiac lesions: Endocardial cushion defects (ASD)
- Other associated disorders (GIT and Hematological):
  - o Duodenal atresia
  - o AML
  - o CML
- Most common cause of down syndrome: Maternal non-disjunction during meiosis
- Other predictors of Down syndrome:
  - o Short femur length on USG
  - o Increased maternal serum hCG

Turner syndrome:

- Lymphedema
- Short stature
- Webbed neck
- Low posterior hairline
- Cubitus valgus (increased carrying angle)
- Coarctation of aorta
- Short 4th metacarpal
- Karyotype: 45 XO

Late congenital syphilis:

- Hutchinson's triad:
  - o Hutchinson teeth
  - o 8th cranial nerve deafness
  - o Interstitial keratitis
- Best to diagnose congenital syphilis: IgM FTA-ABS

Perinatal syphilis:

- Treponema can cross placenta any time but do not attack fetus before 16 weeks
- Rate of transmission is highest (50%) if mother is in secondary stage of syphilis

IV. DISORDERS OF CARDIOVASCULAR SYSTEM

Right to left shunts:

- TOF
- TGV
- Tricuspid atresia

Atrial septal defect:

- ASD + Bony abnormalities: Holt Oram syndrome
- Most common type defect: Ostium secundum (50-70%) located in fossa ovalis
- Usually asymptomatic
- Prophylaxis for infective endocarditis is not indicated
- Spontaneous closure may occur in first 4 years of life (40%)
- Non-surgical/device (closure by Clamshell and amplatzer) is needed if the pulmonary to systemic blood flow ratio is >1.5:1

Patent ductus arteriosus/PDA:

- Persistent duct between the left pulmonary artery and the descending aorta (5-10 mm distal to the origin of subclavian artery)
- Seen in rubella
- Closure is done by: Prostaglandin inhibitor
- Patient is asymptomatic in small PDA
- A large PDA causes lower respiratory tract infection, atelectasis and congestive heart failure
- PDA does not close spontaneously in full term infants

- Congestive heart failure and recurrent pneumonia develops if shunt is large. Small PDA may predispose to bacterial endocarditis
- Management: Prophylaxis of bacterial endocarditis
- Non-surgical closure by Rashkind PDA occlusion device
- Anatomical existence of PDA is an indication for surgery regardless of size

Coarctation of aorta:

- Most common site: Most common below origin of left subclavian artery
- Upper extremity hypertension
- Lower extremity hypotension
- Dizziness

Tetralogy of Fallot:

- Features:
    - o VSD
    - o Pulmonary stenosis
    - o Over-riding of aorta
    - o Right ventricular hypertrophy
- Most common cyanotic heart disease
- Most common symptom: Exercise intolerance and dyspnea on exertion
- Right to left shunt
- Most patients are symptomatic by 6-12 months of age
- Cyanosis and congestive cardiac failure may develop
- Older children may show clubbing, polycythemia, hemoptysis etc.
- Management:
    - o Cyanotic/blue/tet spells: Knee-chest position
    - o Classic Blalock-Taussig shunt: Between ipsilateral subclavian artery and pulmonary artery

V. CHILDHOOD MALIGNANCIES

***Retinoblastoma*:**

- Most common inherited malignancy: Retinoblastoma
- Most common primary ocular tumor of childhood
- 90% cases diagnosed by 3-4 years
- Second neoplasms are a major concern
    - o Osteosarcoma is the most common 2nd malignancy

Neuroblastoma:

- Most common malignant neoplasm in infancy: Neuroblastoma
- Most common presentation: Large abdominal mass
- Metastasizes to: Bone (facial bones, skull) most commonly
- Most common intra-abdominal and extracranial solid tumor in children
- Malignant tumor of autonomic nervous system arising from the neural crest
- Disease of early childhood
- 90% of patients present within 5 years
- 50% present within first 2 years of life
- Most common site of primary tumors is the adrenal gland

Wilm's tumour:

- Also known as: Nephroblastoma
- Most common presenting symptom: Palpable abdominal mass
- Most common malignant tumor of the kidney
- 80% of the patients present within 5 years of age
- Peak age at diagnosis is 2-3 years
- Presents as asymptomatic abdominal mass
- Other features: Hematuria, hypertension, abdominal pain

VI. JAUNDICE

Jaundice:

- Physiological jaundice appears on: 3rd day (clinically undetectable after 14th day)
- Most common cause of jaundice within 24 hours after birth:
    - o Erythroblastosis fetalis/Hemolytic disease of the newborn
    - o More severe if Rh incompatibility
    - o ABO incompatibility is most common type
- Other causes of neonatal hyperbilirubinemia in <24 hours:
    - o Deficiency of G-6-PD
    - o Hereditary spherocytosis

- o Homozygous alpha thalassemia
- Breast milk jaundice is due to: Pregnandiole
- Kernicterus: Unconjugated bilirubin deposited in basal ganglia

Breast milk jaundice:

- It presents as prolonged unconjugated hyperbilirubinemia
- Develops after 72 hours, peaks at 10-14 days (18 mg%) and subsides by 6-10 weeks
- Conjugation of bilirubin in liver is compromised because of presence of 3-alpha-20-beta pregnanediol
- Urine is pale colorless
- Golden yellow stools

Physiological jaundice:

- Rise in level of bilirubin in physiological jaundice: Less than 5 mg/dl/day
- Incidence: 70% in preterm; 60% in term. Time to appear: Always after 24 hours in preterm; 36-72 hours in term
- Peak of jaundice: 5-7 days in preterm; 4-6 days in term
- Maximum bilirubin level reached: 15 mg% in preterm; 12 mg% in term
- Clearance of jaundice: <14 days in preterm; 10 days in term
- No treatment required

VII. DISORDERS OF GASTROINTESTINAL TRACT

Infantile hypertrophic pyloric stenosis/IHPS:

- Age at presentation: Appears around within a month after birth
- Metabolic abnormality: Hypokalemic metabolic alkalosis
- Compensated by: Paradoxical aciduria

Intussusception:

- Most common cause of intestinal obstruction in children: Intussusception (in neonate, it is duodenal atresia)
- Gross examination abdomen: Sausage shaped periumbilical mass
- Appearance of stools: Red currant jelly stools

VIII. DISORDERS OF HEMATOPOIETIC SYSTEM

Anemia:

- Hypochromic, microcytic anemia with decreased serum iron and raised TIBC: Iron deficiency anemia
- Hypochromic, microcytic anemia with increased serum ferritin and decreased TIBC: Anemia of chronic diseases

Iron deficiency anemia:

- Microcytic hypochromic RBCs
- Low:
  - o MCV
  - o Myeloid: erythroid ratio
  - o Serum iron
  - o Serum ferritin
  - o RBC protoporphyrin
- Raised: TIBC
- Most common type of anemia in children: IDA
- First indicator of response after iron therapy: Increased reticulocyte count
- Begins to appear in 3-4 days, with a peak of 10 days after initiation of treatment
- An increase in hemoglobin by 0.5-1 gm% is an optimum response to iron therapy
- Iron therapy should be continued for 1-3 months for treatment of IDA and further 2-3 months, to replenish the iron stores
- Early indicator of iron deficiency anemia: Low Serum ferritin

Thalassemia:

- Beta thalassemia is quantitative defect in hemoglobin synthesis
- There is reduced synthesis of beta-globin chain with normal alpha-chain
- Spleen size: Splenomegaly
- Facies: Hemolytic/chipmunk facies

- Osmotic fragility: Decreased
- Skull X-ray: Hair on end appearance
- Diagnostic test: Electrophoresis
- In beta-thalassemia major (Hemoglobin: <5 gm%):
  - o HbF: 50-96% (normally traces after 1 year of age)
  - o HbA2: 4-10% (normally 2-3%)
  - o HbA: 0% (normally 90%)
- In beta-thalassemia minor/carrier state (Hemoglobin level: 10-12 gm%):
  - o HbF: 1-5%
  - o HbA2: 4-9%
- Absence of HbA and elevation of HbF suggest thalassemia major
- Presence of elevated HbA2 alone suggests the diagnosis of thalassemia trait
- Peripheral blood smear:
  - o Microcytosis and hypochromia
  - o Target cells

IX. DISORDERS OF GENITOURINARY SYSTEM

Vesicoureteral reflux/VUR:

- Most common cause of renal scarring in children: VUR
- Straining and dribbling of urine in a male child with recurrent UTI
- Diagnosis is by: MCUG

Nephrotic syndrome:

- Most common cause of nephrotic syndrome in children: Minimal change disease
- Proteinuria value: More than 3.5 gm/day
- Albumin: Hypoalbuminemia (<2.5 g/dL) leading to edema
- Lipids: Hyperlipidemia leading to lipiduria
- Coagulation status: Hypercoagulability
- Most common sign is massive edema

For better preparation and success in AIIMS-NORCET Exam, download **'drkamalkvgroup'** mobile app from Google Playstore.

WhatsApp: +91 84 7000 4333

X. INBORN ERRORS OF METABOLISM

Glycogen storage diseases:

- Von Gierkes disease is due to deficiency of: Glucose-6-phosphatase deficiency
- Andersen disease is due to deficiency of: Branching enzyme
- McArdles disease is due to deficiency of: Muscle phosphorylase

Galactosemia:

- Autosomal recessive
- Galactosemia is due to deficiency of: GPUT/galactose-1-phosphate-uridyl transferase
- Accumulation of galactilol/dulcitol produces cataract
- Lactose free diet and early restriction of all type of milk

Phenylketonuria:

- Deficiency of: Phenyl-Alanine Hydroxylase (type I)/Its cofactor BH4 tetrahydro-biopterin (type II and III)
- Mental retardation
- Myoclonic seizures
- Vomiting
- Eczematous skin rash
- Hyperactivity etc.
- Urine odour: Musty/mousy odour (due to phenylacetic acid)
- Management:
  - o Lifelong low phenylalanine diet
  - o Tyrosine supplementation (tyrosine becomes essential)

Homocystinuria:

- Enzyme deficient in homocystinuria: Cystathionine synthetase
- Most characteristic feature: Subluxation of the ocular lens
- Treatment: Large doses of pyridoxine (100-500 mg/day)

Other conditions:

- Urine turns dark on standing in: Alkaptonuria (deficiency of homogentisate oxidase)

- Enzyme deficient in Maple syrup urine disease: Branched chain alpha ketoacid dehydrogenase

XI. DISORDERS OF NERVOUS SYSTEM

Meningitis

- Most common presentation of neonatal meningitis: Poor breastfeeding
- Most common cause (in neonates) of bacterial meningitis:
  - o Group B streptococci (Worldwide)
  - o E. coli (India)
- Causes of aseptic meningitis: Mumps virus, polio virus etc.

Febrile seizures:

- Most common cause of seizure in newborn: Hypoxic ischemic encephalopathy
- Most common type of seizure in newborn: Subtle

For better preparation and success in AIIMS-NORCET Exam, download **'drkamalkvgroup'** mobile app from Google Playstore.

WhatsApp: +91 84 7000 4333

XII. DISORDERS OF ENDOCRINE SYSTEM

Congenital hypothyroidism:

- Posterior fontanelle: Large and open
- Social smile and eyebrows: Absent
- Development:
  - o Growth retardation
  - o Delayed puberty
- Temperature: Cold extremities
- Effect on physiological jaundice: Prolongation

For better preparation and success in AIIMS-NORCET Exam, download **'drkamalkvgroup'** mobile app from Google Playstore.

WhatsApp: +91 84 7000 4333

4 CHAPTER Community Health Nursing

I. BIOSTATISTICS

Mean:

- Calculated as sum of all values divided by the total number of values
- For example, mean of 2, 3 and 4 would be calculated as:
  - o Take sum of 2, 3 and 4. This is 9
  - o Divide it by total number of values. These are 3
  - o 9 ÷ 3 equals to 3

Mode:

- It is the most frequently occurring value
- For example, mode of 2, 3, 4, 3 would be 3 as 3 is coming twice in the given set of numbers

Median:

- In ascending/descending order, the middle most value is the median if total numbers of value are odd (average of middle two values in case of even numbers)
- For example, median of 2, 4, 3 would be 3 (by arranging the values in ascending order as 2, 3, 4 or in descending order as 4, 3, 2)

Standard deviation/SD:

- 95% of values fall under: 2SD
- SD is most appropriate measure of dispersion
- SD is calculated as the RMS (root mean square) deviation of the values from the mean

Sample registration system:

- SRS is essentially a dual record system for providing quick and reliable estimates of birth and death rates on a continuous basis at national and state level separately for rural and urban areas
- An independent half-yearly survey of births and deaths by an investigator is done

Bar diagrams/Charts

- It is a simple diagram or a chart, popularly used to compare the magnitude of the qualitative data
- Bars are the rectangles drawn along the graph sheet

SAMPLING

Simple random sampling:

- Sample is drawn in such a way that each unit has an equal chance of being drawn in a sample
- Method includes lottery method, computer software etc.

Stratified random sampling:

- Population is divided to groups/classes and sample is drawn from each group at random

Cluster random sampling:

- Basically, used for assessing immunization status of children under immunization
- 30 clusters, each containing 7 children (30 × 7 technique; total of 210 children)

II. NUTRITION

Proteins:

- Protein Efficiency Ratio: Weight gain (in grams) per gram of protein intake
- Digestibility coefficient/DC: Ratio of Nitrogen absorbed to Nitrogen consumed
- Biological value/BV: Ratio of Nitrogen retained to Nitrogen absorbed
- Net Protein Utilization: Product of BV and DC

Xerophthalmia:

- Most common in aged 1-3 years
- First clinical symptom of vitamin A deficiency: Night blindness/nyctalopia
- Under National immunization schedule, 1 lac IU is given at 9 months of age (along with measles vaccine)

VITAMINS

Vitamin A:

- Earliest symptom of vitamin A deficiency: Night blindness/ Nyctalopia
- Earliest sign of vitamin A deficiency: Conjunctival xerosis (characteristic appearance of 'emerging like sand banks at receding tide')
- Effect of fat on absorption of vitamin A: Increases
- Vitamin A deficiency is a child health problem if prevalence of night blindness in children's aged 6 months to 6 years is: 1%
- For Bitot's spots the prevalence should be more than >0.5%

Other vitamins:

- Vitamin which prevents lipid peroxidation: Vitamin E (also vitamin A and vitamin C)
- Vitamin which is required for gamma carboxylation: Vitamin K

Iron-Folic acid supplementation:

- During pregnancy, IFA tablets contain (specific protection): 100 mg elemental iron and 500 microgram of FA (daily)
- Amount for paediatric population (under RCH): Amount is 1/5th (20 mg elemental iron and 100 microgram of FA daily)

Egg:

- Poor in: Carbohydrate, Vitamin C
- Energy yielded from egg: 70 Kcal
- Net Protein Utilization/NPU of hen's egg: 96

Milk:

- Skimmed milk: Fat has been removed from the milk
- Milk is a poor source of: Iron and vitamin C
- Pasteurization of milk: Rapidly heating milk, then keeping it uniformly and then allowing it to cool rapidly
- Pasteurization kills: 90% of bacteria in milk, including heat resistant tubercle bacillus and Q fever
- Pasteurization doesn't kill: Thermoduric bacteria, nor the bacterial spores
- Methods of pasteurization of milk:
    - Holder/Vat method (used for small and rural communities)
    - HTST method (Most widely done procedure)
    - HHST method
    - UHT method
- Tests for pasteurization of milk to check adequacy:
    - Phosphatase test (widely test)
    - Standard plate count
    - Coliform count
- Use of pasteurization: Milk can be preserved for 8 to 12 hours at 18 degree C
- Methylene blue reduction test/MBRT in milk is done to:
    - Detection of micro-organism in the milk/contamination of milk
    - MBRT is carried out on milk accepted for pasteurization

Cereals:

- Jaggery has high concentration of: Iron
- Ragi, dates are rich source of: Calcium
- Pulses are deficient in: Methionine (and cysteine)
- Cereals are deficient in: Threonine (and Lysine)
- Maize is deficient in: Tryptophan (and Lysine)
- Highest biological value is: Egg

FATTY ACID/FA

Essential FA:

- Most important EFA is linoleic acid as it serve as a basis of production of EFA
- Deficiency of EFA lead to phrenoderma/toad skin
- Example of EFA (cannot be synthesized in human body and hence to be supplied in diet):
    - o Linoleic acid (PUFA)
    - o Linolenic acid (PUFA)
    - o Arachidonic acid
    - o Eicosapentanoic acid
    - o Not all EFA are PUFA (polyunsaturated fatty acids)

Rich source of linoleic acid:

- Safflower oil (73%)
- Corn oil (57%)
- Sunflower oil (56%)
- Soyabean oil (51)

Endemic fluorosis:

- Mottling of dental enamel, with chalky white appearance (Caries) best seen on upper jaw incisors at level more than 1.5 ppm
- Skeletal fluorosis at fluorine level between 3-6 ppm
- Intervention: Nalgonda technique (NEERI, Nagpur). It involves addition of lime, alum and bleaching powder followed by flocculation, sedimentation and filtration

FOOD ADULTERATION

Epidemic dropsy:

- Epidemic dropsy is due to contamination of mustard oil with: Argemone oil (containing sanguinarine)
- Biochemical Effect of sanguinarine: Interferes with oxidation of pyruvic acid, which accumulates in blood
- This lead to sudden non-inflammatory edema of lower limbs (bilateral), diarrhoea, glaucoma, cardiac failure, dyspnea and death

Aflatoxicosis:

- Toxin: Aflatoxin
- Foodstuff affected by: Aspergillus flavus

Ergotism:

- Toxin: Clavine alkaloids
- Foodstuff affected by: Claviceps fusiformis

Lathyrism:

- Toxin: Beta-Oxayl Amino Alanine/BOAA
- Foodstuff (Kesari dal) affected by: Lathyrus sativus

III. ENVIRONMENT

Sound:

- Hearing ability is measured by: Audiometer
- Tympanic membrane ruptures if the intensity of sound is more than: 150 -160 dB
- Maximum tolerable limit of sound per day is: 85 – 90 dB

Air:

- Chemical indicators of air pollution:
    - o Coefficient of haze
    - o Smoke and soiling index
    - o Best indicator is Sulphur dioxide

Water:

- Recommended fluorine concentration in water: 0.5 – 0.8 ppm (<1.5 ppm)
- Fluoride concentration: 1.5 mg/L

Drinking water quality standards:

- E. coli or thermotolerant coliforms: Nil
- Nitrites (recent contamination): <3 mg/L
- Nitrates (remote contamination): <50 mg/L

IV. HEALTH CARE IN INDIA

Health care in India:

- Tertiary level of care: Medical Colleges and Hospitals

- Secondary level of care: Community health centre
- Primary level of care: Primary health centre
- Subcenter

ASHA:

- Works under NRHM mission
- Educated till VIII class

MPW:

- Multipurpose worker is present at Subcentre
- Caters to a population of 5000

VHG:

- 1 village health guide caters to a population of: 1000 rural population (Trained Birth Attendant/TBA, Anganwadi worker/AWW also caters to a population of 1000)
- Preferably female
- Educated upto at least VI class (same qualification for TBA, AWW, MPW)
- Trained at PHC (200 hours in 3 months)

PHC:

- Population covered by PHC in hilly/tribal area is: 20,000 (30,000 in plains)
- PHC has 4-6 beds
- Referral centre for 6 subcentres
- 1-2 medical officers (total staff of 15)
- Under NTCP, PHC is said to be PHC-R if: Microscopy + Radiology facility exist

Subcenter:

- 1 subcenter caters to a population of: 5,000 in plain areas (3000 in hilly/tribal area)
- Number of staff: 3
- Most peripheral and first contact point between community and health care system

TBA:

- A trained birth dai/trained birth attendant caters to a population of: 1000 (rural population)
- Training at PHC, subcentre or MCH centre for 30 days (has to conduct 2 supervised deliveries)
- Duty includes conducting home deliveries in aseptic manner

Community Health Centers:

- As per RCH, first referral unit is: CHC
- Number of beds in CHC: 30
- Referral centre for 4 PHCs
- Total staff of 30-13 including 4 specialists (physician, surgeon, pediatrician and gynecologist)

V. INTERNATIONAL HEALTH

Important days:

- 1st December: World AIDS day
- 1st July: Doctors day
- 31st May: No Tobacco day

UNICEF (United Nations Children Fund):

- Headquarter: New York, USA
- Established in: 1946

UNESCO:

- Headquarter: Paris

FAO (Food and Agricultural Organization):

- Headquarter: Rome, Italy

WHO:

- Headquarter: Geneva, Switzerland
- Founded on: 7th April, 1948 (celebrated as World Health Day)

VI. HEALTH PROGRAMMES

ICDS Scheme (Integrated Child Development Services):

- Launched in the year: 1975
- Beneficiaries in ICDS:
  - o Women in reproductive age group
  - o Pregnant and lactating women
  - o Children below 6 years of age
- Focal point of delivery of ICDS: Anganwadi

IMNCI/Integrated Management of Neonatal and Childhood Illness:

- Beneficiaries:
  - o Infants (2 months) to 5 years children
  - o Newborn and young infants (under 2 months of age)

NVBDCP (National Vector Borne Disease Control Programme):

- Launched in the year: 2003-2004
- VBD includes:
  - o Malaria
  - o Dengue/Dengue Hemorrhagic fever
  - o Chikungunya
  - o Filaria
  - o Kala azar
  - o Japanese encephalitis

NIDDCP/National Iodine Deficiency Disorders Control Programme:

- NGCP/National Goitre Control Programme was launched in the year: 1962
- NGCP was renamed as NIDDCP in the year: 1992
- Level of iodization in salt at production level: 30 parts per million
- Level of iodization in salt at production level: 15 ppm

NLCP (National Leprosy Control Programme):

- Launched in: 1955
- Aims to control leprosy through:
  - o Monotherapy with Dapsone
  - o Early detection of cases

NLEP (National Leprosy Elimination Programme):

- Launched in: 1983

NPCB (National Programme for Control of Blindness):

- Launched in 1976 as 100% centrally funded programme
- NPCB cut-off for blindness: <6/60
- National Institute of Ophthalmology (AIIMS) is the apex institute
- Under National Programme for Control of Blindness, vision screening for children is conducted by: School teachers
- WHO definition of blindness: Visual acuity of less than 3/60 in better eye with best possible correction (BEBPC)
- Most common cause of blindness in India: Cataract

NACP/National Aids Control Programme:

- Launched in the year:
  - o Phase I in 1992
  - o Phase II in 1999
  - o Phase III in 2007

VII. CONTRACEPTION

IUCD (Intrauterine Uterine Contraceptive Device):

- IUCD components and their effects:
  - o Copper: Affects cervical mucus making sperm motility, capacitation and survival difficult
  - o Hormones: Cervical mucus viscosity increased which prevents sperm entry into cervix. Interferes with implantation
  - o Foreign body reaction reducing chances of fertilization
- CuT 200 is inserted post-natally after: 8 weeks
- If CuT 200 is implanted in myometrium, treatment is: Hysteroscopic removal
- Complications of IUCD:
  - o Most common is bleeding
  - o Second most common side effect is pain (which requires removal of IUCD)
  - o Pelvic inflammatory disease
  - o Pregnancy with IUCD in situ
  - o Ectopic pregnancy (highest with progestasert)
  - o Uterine perforation
  - o Spontaneous expulsion

Cu-T 380A:

- 380 represents surface area of copper (mm^2)
- 'A' represents silver or gold (with copper)
- CuT 380A should be replaced after every: 10 years (Others have a life of 3-5 years)

Oral Contraceptive Pills/OCP:

- OCP of choice in lactating females: Minipill/progesterone only pill

- After discontinuing OCP, fertility returns after: 6 months
- Adverse effects of OCPs (ABCDEFGHI):
  - o **A**ltered lipid profile
  - o **B**lood clotting/thrombosis (cerebral/venous), breast tenderness
  - o **C**arcinoma (breast, cervix), Cholestatic jaundice
  - o **D**epression
  - o **E**levated BP (hypertension)
  - o **F**luid retention (weight gain)
  - o **G**allbladder disease
  - o **H**epatocellular adenoma
  - o **I**nfarction (myocardial)
- Beneficial effects of OCPs (EUROPE):
  - o **E**ctopic pregnancy
  - o **U**terine/endometrial carcinoma
  - o **R**educed chances of Iron deficiency anemia
  - o **O**varian (benign) disease/ovarian cysts and ovarian (malignant) disease (ovarian carcinoma)
  - o **P**ID
  - o **E**ndometriosis
- Absolute contraindications for OCPs (ACTH):
  - o **A**bnormal uterine bleeding (undiagnosed)
  - o **C**ancer (breast and genital)
  - o **T**hromboembolism
  - o **H**epatic diseases

NORPLANT (Levonorgestrel):

- Subdermal implant
- 6 silastic capsules containing 35 mg levonorgestrel each
- Effective for 5 years
- Mechanism of action: Prevents ovulation

STERILIZATION

Criteria for sterilization:

- Age of male between 25-50 years and
- Age of female between 20-45 years
- Couple should have at least 2 living children at the time of operation

Pomeroy's method of female sterilization:

- Isthmoampullary portion is ligated (middle portion is formed into a loop which is tied with catgut and excised)

NSV (non-scalpel vasectomy)/key-hole vasectomy:

- Vas is taken out through a small puncture wound and no stitches are needed after the procedure
- Surgical hook (and not scalpel) is used to enter scrotum

EMERGENCY CONTRACEPTION

Emergency contraception is by:

- OCP (Combined OCPs/Minipills)
- CuT (must be inserted within 5 days)
- Levonorgesterol

Dosage for emergency contraception:

- OCPs with 30 microgram estrogen (4 pills immediately followed by 4 more pills after 12 hours)
- OCPs with 50 microgram estrogen (2 pills followed by 2 more pills 12 hours later)
- Minipill 75 mg (has to be taken within 72 hours)
- Mifepristone RU 486/antiprogestin (600 mg stat within 72 hours)

Pearl Index:

- Studying effectiveness of contraception
- It is number of failures per 100 woman years (HWY) of exposure
- Calculated as:

$$\frac{\text{Total accidental pregnancies} \times 1200}{\text{Total months of exposure}}$$

VIII. VACCINES

Properties of an ideal vaccine:

- It should be stable, cheap and safe
- It should require few administrations to produce immunity
- It should be effective in all age groups
- It should be able to pass maternal immunity to fetus as well
- It should produce immunity rapidly
- It should be effective against all variants of the micro-organism
- It should provide life-long immunity

Cold chain:

- System of transportation and storage of vaccines from the point of manufacturer to the place of administration
- In India, cold chain is maintained at: +2 to +8 degree C temperature

VACCINATION

Features of live vaccines:

- Long duration of immunity
- Contains major and minor antigen
- Live vaccines are prepared from live attenuated organisms
- Single dose is sufficient to attain immunity (except oral polio virus)

Examples of live vaccine:

- BCG
- Yellow fever (17D)
- MMR
- Typhoral/Ty21A
- Oral polio
- Epidemic typhus
- Chickenpox

Examples of killed vaccine:

- Salk polio
- Pertussis
- Rabies
- KFD
- Killed influenza
- JE
- HBV
- Typhim Vi
- Meningococcal
- Cholera

Cell fraction/Fragment derived vaccine:

- Hepatitis B (polypeptides)
- Meningococcal vaccine (polysaccharide antigen of cell wall)
- Pneumococcal vaccine (polysaccharide capsule)

Toxoids:

- Tetanus toxoid
- Diphtheria toxoid

Freeze dried vaccine:

- Yellow fever (should be used within 30 minutes)
- Measles (should be used within 1-4 hours)
- BCG (should be used within 3 hours)

Reconstituted vaccines:

- BCG
- Measles
- Yellow fever

Other important facts:

- Ring immunization: Given around 100 yards of a case detected
- BCG (live attenuated vaccine) is given: Intradermally
- TY21 A (vaccine) is given for: Typhoid
- Influenza vaccine is administered as: Nose drops
- HPV vaccine is: Both bivalent and quadrivalent

Vaccine and strains:

- BCG: Danish 1331
- OPV: Sabin strain
- Chickenpox: Oka strain
- Measles: Edmonston Zagreb/Schwartz/Moraten strains
- Mumps: Jeryll Lyn/Leningrad/L-Zagreb/Urabe
- Rubella: RA-27/3
- Yellow fever: 17 D
- JE: Nakayama

Contraindications of vaccines:

- All live vaccines are C/I in pregnancy except Yellow fever
- Symptomatic HIV: All live vaccines are C/I except BCG and MMR (None of the vaccine is C/I in asymptomatic HIV)
- All live vaccines are C/I in immune-suppressive and cortico-steroid therapy

Vaccine C/I in pregnancy:

- MMR (live vaccines)
- Yellow fever, though contraindicated can be given under special circumstances

Supportive in vaccines:

- Preservative in DPT: Thiomersal
- Adsorbant used in DPT: Aluminium phosphate/Aluminium hydroxide
- Preservative in Measles vaccine: Neomycin and erythromycin
- Thermostabilizer in OPV: $MgCl_2$

IMPORTANT VACCINES

OPV:

- Dose and route: 2 drops are given orally
- Given at: 6, 10 and 14 weeks

BCG:

- Dose: 0.5 ml is intradermally at left shoulder
- Given at: Birth

DPT:

- Dose and route: 0.5 ml intramuscular in lateral part of thigh
- Given at: 6, 10 and 14 weeks

Measles:

- Dose and route: 0.5 ml, subcutaneous
- Given at: 9 months

Hepatitis B:

- Dose and route: 0.5 ml, intramuscular
- Given at: 0, 1 and 6 months as per IAP (Indian Academy of Pediatrics); 6, 10 and 14 weeks as per NIS (National Immunization Schedule)

Heat sensitivity of vaccines:

- Storage temperature for most of the vaccines: +2 degree C to 8 degree C
- OPV is highly heat sensitive vaccine (should be kept in freezer; -20 degree C)
- Vaccine vial monitors (VVM) are used for potency testing of OPV

Reverse cold chain:

- Maintenance of optimum cold temperature during transport of vaccine from periphery to the laboratory for potency testing as in OPV
- Also useful for transport of stool samples

IX. STERILIZATION AND DISINFECTION

Physical methods of sterilization:

- Sunlight and drying
- Dry heat
  - o Flaming
  - o Incineration
  - o Hot air oven
- Moist heat
  - o Less than 100 degree C
  - o More than 100 degree C
- Radiation
  - o Non-ionizing: Infrared rays, Ultraviolet rays
  - o Ionizing: Gamma rays, X-rays
- Filtration
  - o Candle filter
  - o Asbestos/Seitz filter
  - o Millipore filter

Chemical methods of sterilization:

- Phenol
- Alcohol
- Aldehyde
  - o Formaldehyde
  - o Glutaraldehyde
- Halogens
  - o Chlorine
  - o Iodine
- Ethylene oxide: For sterilization of sutures, heart-lung machines etc.
- Quarternary ammonium compounds

Sterilization:

- Sterilization is a process by an article is made free of all living organisms including spores.

Disinfection:

- Disinfection is a process by which a non-living object is made free of all pathogenic organisms, but non-pathogenic organisms and spores are left behind

Bacteriostatic agent:

- Agent, added to colony, inhibits growth and vice versa

Cidex:

- Endoscopes, rubber/plastic tubes, face masks and corrugated tubes are sterilized by: Glutaraldehyde
- Cidex is: 2% glutaraldehyde

Other important points about sterilization:

- Disposable syringes are sterilized by: Gamma rays, Ethylene oxide
- Cold sterilization is by (Sterilize without increasing temperature): Gamma rays, X-rays and cosmic rays
- Vaccines are sterilized by: Heat inactivation
- Hospital dressings are best disposed of by: Incinerator (not done for sharp)
- Reidel walker coefficient: Determines germicidal efficiency of disinfectants (as compared to phenol)

Autoclaving:

- Bacterial spores are destroyed by: Autoclaving
- Attain temperature of 122 degree C under 15 lb/sq inch pressure for 15 minutes
- Most effective for killing spores
- Used for linen, bedsheets, dressings, gloves, OT appliances, most of culture media
- Not suitable for plastic and sharp instrument
- Bacillus stearothermophilus is sterilization control

Hot air oven:

- Utilizes 180 degree C for 1 hour
- Used for lab glasswares/glass syringes, test tubes, surgical instruments (sharp)
- Liquid paraffin, dusting powder
- It may destroy plastic/rubber objects (mattresses)
- Biological control for adequacy of sterilization: Spores of bacillus subtilis

Formaldehyde:

- Liquid form is used for preserving anatomical specimens
- Gaseous form is employed for fumigation of operation theatres

Glutaraldehye:

- Sterilization of endoscopes, bronchoscopes and cystoscope
- Sterilization of face mask and endotracheal tube

X. COMMUNICABLE DISEASES

Cleans of safe delivery:

- Employed for: Elimination of neonatal tetanus
- CLEANS include:
  - o Clean delivery surface
  - o Clean hands (birth attendants)
  - o Clean cord cut (blade/instrument)
  - o Clean cord tie
  - o Clean cord stump (no applicant)

Smallpox/variola

- India declared free of smallpox in: April 1977
- WHO declared eradication of smallpox on: 08/05/1980

Typhoid/enteric fever:

- Causative agent: Salmonella typhii
- Mode of transmission: Feco-oral
- Laboratory tests (BASU)
  - o 1st week: Blood culture
  - o 2nd week: Antibodies
  - o 3rd week: Stool culture
  - o 4th week: Urine test
- Features: Pea-soup diarrhea
- Treatment:
  - o Cases: Quinolones (Ciprofloxacin)
  - o Carriers: Ampicillin

Chickenpox:

- Incubation period/IP: 14-16 days
- Infectivity of chickenpox lasts for:
  - o 1 day before rash
  - o 6 days after onset of rash
- Features: Rash is pleomorphic (all stages of the rash, i.e., papules, pustules, vesicles may be present at one time)
- Reactivation occurs in 10-30% results in Shingles/Herpes zoster (Shingles is the most common late complication)

- Secondary attack rate: 90%
- Don't give Aspirin: Risk of Reye's syndrome

Diphtheria:

- Incubation Period: 2-6 days
- Caused by: Corynebacterium diphtheria
- Mode of infection: Droplet infection
- For susceptibility: Schick test

Measles/rubeola:

- Caused by: RNA paramyxo virus (measles virus)
- Special feature in oral cavity: Koplik's spot
- Incubation period: 10 days (range 10-14 days)
- Rash appears on:
  - o 4th day after onset of fever
  - o 14th day from exposure
- Period of communicability: 4th day before rash to 5 days before rash
- Rare complication of measles: SSPE
- Protective effect of measles vaccine is exerted within: 11-12 days after administration and persist throughout life
- Contamination of measles vaccine can cause/same vial is used after 4 hours: TSS (toxic shock syndrome)
- Features: It shows cyclical trend (cases occur every 2-3 years)
- Measles virus cannot survive outside human body
- Secondary attack rate: >80%
- No carriers
- For eradication: 95% of population must be vaccinated
- Most common complication: Otitis media

Cholera:

- IP: 1-2 days
- Caused by: Vibrio cholera
- Feature: Rice water stool
- Essential part of treatment: Oral Rehydration Solution
- Chemoprophylaxis: Tetracycline
- Drug of choice in adults: Doxycyline
- Drug of choice in children: Cotrimoxazole
- Drug of choice in pregnancy: Furazolidone

Rubella:

- Incubation period: 14-21 days
- Risk to fetus is maximum if mother gets infected during: 6-12 weeks of pregnancy
- Congenital rubella syndrome:
  - o Deafness (most common if mother affected in second trimester)
  - o Cardiac malformations/PDA (most common if mother is affected in first trimester)
  - o Cataracts
- Recommended vaccination strategy to prevent congenital rubella syndrome:
  - o 15-34/39 years women
  - o Interrupt transmission of rubella by vaccinating all children 1-14 years
  - o All children under 1 years of age
- Caused by ssRNA virus (Rubivirus)
- Mild rashes noticed on 3rd day of fever (3rd day measles) and characteristic posterior auricular, posterior cervical and occipital adenitis
- Forchheimers spots: Discrete rose coloured spots over soft palate
- Secondary attack rate: 90%

Rabies/Hydrophobia:

- Symptoms appear in: About 10 days (4 days – 8 weeks)
- IP Depends on:
  - o Site of bite
  - o Severity of the bite
  - o Number of wounds
  - o Amount of virus injected
  - o Species of biting animal
  - o Protection provided by clothing and treatment taken
- Test used for diagnosing Rabies: Antigen detection using immunoflourescence of skin biopsy
- Vaccine recommended by WHO: HDC vaccine should be replaced by cultures of animal cell lines (fetal bovine kidney, chick embryo fibroblast)
- Post exposure schedule (cell culture vaccine): HDC vaccine
  - o For unimmunized: 6 doses
    - – 0, 3, 7, 14, 28 days
    - – Booster on 90th day
  - o For immunized:
    - – 0, 3 and 7 days
- Pre-exposure:
  - o HDCV 1 ml given as I/M injection
  - o 0,7 and 28 days

- Caused by: Lyssavirus type I
- In 80% of cases, pain and tingling at the site of bite is the only symptom
- Exaggerated reflexes with hydrophobia (pathognomonic)
- Rabies is not seen in Andaman-Nicobar and Lakshwadeep
- Neutralizing antibodies are present in serum/CSF after 8th day (considered as an index of protection against infection with rabies virus)
- Dead end infection
- Street virus:
  - o Naturally occurring cases of Rabies
  - o Incubation period: 20-60 days
  - o Long and variable incubation period
  - o Forms Negri bodies
  - o Multiplication in extra-neural tissues
  - o Not used for vaccine production
- Fixed virus:
  - o Incubation period: 4-6 days
  - o Negri bodies are not formed
  - o Used for vaccine production

Polio:

- IM injections and tonsillectomy should be avoided during polio epidemic because: Risk of paralytic polio increases
- Cause of death in polio: Respiratory paralysis
- Pulse polio was introduced in India in: 1995
- Pulse polio is given to children below: 5 years
- A country is said to be polio FREE if there is no case confirmed for last: 3 years
- In AFP/acute flaccid paralysis, examination for residual paralysis should be done after: 60 days
- Incubation period/IP: 3-35 days
- P1 virus: Most common cause of epidemics
- P2 virus: Most antigenic and easily eradicable
- P3 virus: Most common cause of vaccine associated paralytic polio
- Infectious material: Oropharyngeal secretions and faeces
- For every clinical case, there are 1000 subclinical cases in children and 75 subclinical cases in adults
- History of fever at onset of paralysis is suggestive of polio
- Recommended method of confirmation of paralytic polio: Isolation of wild polio from stool

Influenza:

- Caused by orthomyxovirus (A, B and C)
- Most common cause of outbreaks/epidemics and only cause of pandemic: Type A
- H1N1: Swine flu
- H5N1: Avian flu/Bird flu
- Cyclical trend
- Incubation Period: 18-72 hours
- Vaccines for influenza:
  - o Live attenuated
  - o Killed (may be associated with Guillain-Barré syndrome)
- Swine flu is caused by: H1N1 virus
- Bird/Avian flu is caused by: H5N1
- Drug of choice /DOC for avian influenza/Bird flu and Swine flu is Oseltamivir/Tamiflu

Hookworm:

- Ancylostoma duodenale and Necator Americana
- Chandler's index: Average number of hookworm eggs/gram of stool
- Hookworm infestation is a major health problem if the Chandler's index is more than: 300
- Hookworm infestation causes deficiency of: Iron (as there is blood loss of 0.03-0.2 ml/worm/day)

HIV:

- Subtype most prevalent in India: C (HIV-I)
- Seroconversion takes: 2-12 weeks
- Most common mode of transmission of HIV: Heterosexual mode (male to female is more)
- Risk of transmission by accidental needle prick: 0.3%
- Retroviral sequence in host cell: RNA-DNA-RNA
- p24 antigen disappears after: 6-8 weeks of HIV infection
- Cells attacked in HIV: CD4 cells
- CD4: CD8 ratio is: Reversed
- Window period: Time period between infection to appearance of antibodies in serum
- During window period, both ELISA and western blot are: Negative
- Most common opportunistic infection in an AIDS patient in world: P. carinii
- Most common opportunistic infection in an AIDS patient in India: Mycobacterium TB
- MTCT (Mother to Child Transmission) can be reduced by: Zidovudine, intrapartum nevirapine and LSCS

Pertussis/Whooping cough:

- Media used: Bordet Gengou
- Incubation Period: 1-2 weeks
- Caused by Bordetella pertussis
- Secondary attack rate: More than 90%
- Mode of transmission: Droplet
- Managed by: Erythromycin

DENGUE

DF/Dengue fever/Breakbone fever:

- Dengue is transmitted by (vector): Aedes aegypti (prefers stagnant water)
- IP: 5-6 days
- High grade fever with chills, muscle and joint pains, intense headache, retro-orbital pain, skin rash

Dengue hemorrhagic fever/DHF:

- IP: 4-6 days
- Moderate to marked thrombocytopenia (<1 lakh/cmm)
- Hemorrhagic manifestations
- Positive tourniquet test (>20 petechiae/sq. inch)
- Hemoconcentration/rising hematocrit
- Plus all features of DF

Dengue shock syndrome:

- Dengue hemorrhagic fever and shock
- Features of shock include low BP, tachycardia, Narrow pulse pressure, cold and clammy skin

MALARIA

Man in malaria:

- Intermediate/secondary host
- Asexual phase
- Schizogony (pre-erythrocytic, erythrocytic and exoerythrocytic)

Other important points:

- Size of RBC is increased in: Vivax malaria
- Infective agent of malaria is: Sporozoite, transmitted through bite of a female anopheline mosquito
- Not seen in peripheral blood smear of falciparum: Schizont

TUBERCULOSIS

Tuberculosis:

- Mycobacterium TB was discovered by: Robert Koch
- Prevalence of TB in community is assessed by: Tuberculin test/Mantoux test
- Standard dose of PPD for Mantoux test: 1 TU
- Ghon focus is related to: Primary pulmonary TB
- Ocular lesion associated with primary TB: Phylectenular conjunctivitis
- Characteristic lesion of primary TB: Fibrocaseous lesion
- Category II of DOTS includes: Previously treated smear positive (relapse, failure, default)
- Defaulter is: Has not taken drugs for more than 2 months consecutively any time after starting treatment
- Case finding in RNTCP is based on: Sputum microscopy
- Sputum smear are stained for AFB with Zeihl Neelson stain
- Other tests:
  - o PCR/NAAT test: Extremely sensitive
  - o BACTEC radiometric system: 95% sensitivity
  - o MMR/mass miniature readiography: Not used now
- DOTS means: Short term treatment under supervision; Alternate day treatment given

Tuberculin test:

- Tuberculin is purified protein derivative
- 0.1 ml of 1TU PPD is injected intradermally on forearm and read after 72 hours
- Estimates prevalence of TB infection
- A positive test (induration >9 mm) indicates past/present exposure/infection by M. tuberculosis
- Prognostic significance

LEPROSY/HANSEN'S DISEASE

Leprosy:

- Spreads by: Droplet infection
- Contact transmission:
  - o Skin to skin contact
  - o Contact with soil/fomites
- Leprosy is a public health problem when prevalence is: 1:10,000

- Elimination level of leprosy: Less than 1 case per 10,000
- India achieved level of elimination of leprosy
- Classification system/index related to leprosy:
  - o Ridley Jopling's classification (BI: Counting number of bacilli in average microscopic fields)
  - o Diagnosis of leprosy under National Leprosy

Elimination Programme/NLEP (Clinical basis):

- PBL (Pauci-Bacillary leprosy): 1-5 skin lesions
- MBL (Multi-Bacillary Leprosy): More than 5 skin lesions

Operational classification (for chemotherapy):

- Paucibacillary: <2 skin lesion
- Multibacillary: >2 skin lesions

MBL:

- Managed by 3 drugs (RDC)
- Duration: 12 months
- Annual follow-up till: 5 years

PBL:

- Managed by 2 drugs (RD)
- Duration: 6 months
- Annual follow-up for: 2 years

Dosage of drugs:

- Rifampicin/R: 600 mg once a month, supervised
- Dapsone/D: 100 mg daily
- Clofazimine/C: 300 mg once a month, supervised

PLAGUE

Plague/Black sickness/Mahamari

- Wild rodents are reservoir of infection
- Infected rodents, fleas and pneumonic plague cases are source of infection
- Rat flea (Xenopsylla cheopsis) is the most efficient vector
- Bite of an infected flea or droplet infection (pneumonic plague) is the mode of transmission
- Most common type of plague is bubonic plague (2-7 days)
- Streptomycin is drug of choice
- Tetracycline is chemoprophylactic agent of choice
- Destruction of rat flea is the most effective way of breaking transmission of plague
- Causative agent of plague: Yersinia pestis (Gram-negative, non-motile, coccobacillus)
- Staining done in a case of plague: Wayson's staining
- Most contagious type of plague: Pneumonic plague (1-2 days)
- Complication of bubonic-septicemic plague
- IP: 1-3 days
- Specific flea index: Average number of fleas of each species/rodent
- Best indicator of potential explosiveness of plague outbreak: Specific flea index

XI. NON-COMMUNICABLE DISEASES

Cancer:

- Most common cancer in males in India: Oropharyngeal cancer
- Most common cancer in males causing death in India and Worldwide: Lung cancer
- Most common cancer in males Worldwide: Lung cancer
- Most common cancer in females in India: Cervical cancer
- Most common cancer in females Worldwide: Breast cancer
- Most common cancer in females causing death in India and Worldwide: Breast cancer

Obesity:

- Indices for obesity:
  - o BMI (Quetlet's index)
  - o BMI = Weight (in Kg)/Height^2 (in metre)
  - o Underweight: <18.5
  - o Normal: 18.5 – 24.99
  - o Overweight: 25 – 29.99
  - o Obesity: >30
- Corpulence index: Height independent index
- Other criteria for assessment of obesity:
  - o Ponderal index
  - o Lorentz formula
  - o Skin fold thickness
  - o Waist circumference and WHR/Waist to hip ratio

- Abdominal fat accumulation is assessed by: Waist/hip ratio
- WHR >0.85 in women suggest obesity
- WHR >1 in men suggest obesity

Ischemic/Coronary Heart Disease:

- Known as modern epidemic
- Modifiable risk factors:
  - o Smoking
  - o High blood pressure
  - o Diabetes
  - o Raised cholesterol (>200 mg/dl)
  - o Lack of exercise
- Non-Modifiable risk factors:
  - o Age
  - o Gender
  - o Positive family history
- Recommendations:
  - o Avoid alcohol consumption
  - o Reduce salt intake
  - o Promote complex carbohydrate consumption in diet
  - o Limitation of dietary cholesterol
  - o Reduction of fat intake

XII. OCCUPATIONAL DISEASES

Factory Act - 1948

- Maximum working hours of 48 hours/week and if overtime, then 60 hours/week
- Children less than 14 years should not be employed

Asbestosis:

- Exposure to: Asbestos dust
- Affects: Base of lungs
- Predisposes to:
  - o Mesothelioma
  - o Bronchogenic cancer
  - o Interstitial fibrosis (Ferruginous body)
  - o Pleural plaque

Bagassosis:

- Inhalation of sugarcane dust/molasses/fibrous residue of sugarcane (bagasse)
- Bagasse blocks bronchioles leading to bronchitis and bronchopneumonia
- Bagassosis is a form of extrinsic allergic alveolitis
- Prevention by 2% Propionic acid
- Thermoactinomyces saccharii causes: Bagassosis

Farmers lung:

- Organism causing Farmers lung: Micropolyspora faeni, Aspergillus fumigates
- Exposure to: Mouldy hay, grain, Straw

Byssinosis:

- Textile industry (cotton fibre)
- Monday fever is associated with: Byssinosis

Silicosis:

- Most common chronic occupational disorder
- Notifiable condition under: Factories Act,1948 and Mines Act, 1952
- Occupation associated with silicosis: Silica dust, mines, tunnels
- 0.5 – 3 micron size are particles are most dangerous
- Affects upper lobe of lung
- Chest X-ray shows egg shell calcification
- No effective treatment
- Patient with silicosis are prone to develop:
  - o TB (silicotuberculosis) and nodular fibrosis
  - o Emphysema
  - o Cor pulmonale/right sided heart failure
- Polarizing microscopy demonstrates birefringent crystals of silica
- Snow storm appearance is seen in: Silicosis

XIII. BIOMEDICAL WASTE MANAGEMENT

COLOURED CONTAINERS, WASTE CATEGORIES AND MODE OF TREATMENT

Red colour container:

- Contaminated waste (recyclable)
- Waste generated from disposable items such as tubing, bottles intravenous tubes and sets, catheters, urine bags, syringes (without needles and fixed needle syringes) and vaccutainers with their needles cut and gloves
- Treated by:
  - o Autoclaving/chemical treatment/microwaving

Yellow colour container:

- Human anatomical waste
- Animal anatomical waste
- Soiled waste
- Expired or discarded medicines
- Chemical wastes
- Chemical liquid waste
- Discarded linen, mattresses, beddings contaminated with blood or body fluids
- Microbiology, biotechnology and other clinical laboratory waste
- Treated by:
  - o Incineration, deep burial

Blue coloured container:

- Glasswares (broken or discarded and contaminated glass including medicine vials and ampoules except those contaminated with cytotoxic waste)
- Metallic body implants
- Treated by:
  - o Autoclaving/microwaving/shredding/chemical treatment and destruction

White coloured container:

- Waste sharps including metals (needles, syringes with fixed needles, needles from needle tip cutter or burner, scalpels, blades or any other contaminated sharp object that may cause puncture and cutes)
- Treated by:
  - o Autoclaving or dry heat sterilization followed by shredding, mutilation or encapsulization in metallic containers or cement concrete

CATEGORIES OF BIOMEDICAL WASTE

Category	Biomedical waste	Includes
1	Human anatomical waste	Human tissues, body parts, organs, placenta
2	Animal waste	Animal tissues, body parts, organs, blood, carcasses, fluids
3	Microbiological and Biotechnology waste	Waste from laboratory cultures, human and animal cell culture used in research, waste from production of biological, toxins, dishes used for transfer of cultures
4	Waste sharp	Needles, scalpels, syringes, blade, glass
5	Discarded medicine and cytotoxic drugs	Waste comprising outdated, contaminated and discarded medicines
6	Soiled waste	Items contaminated with blood and body fluids
7	Solid waste	Waste generated from disposal items other than sharp such as tubings, catheters, intravenous sets etc.
8	Liquid waste	Waste generated from laboratory and washing, cleaning, housekeeping etc.
9	Incineration ash	Ash generated from incineration of any biomedical waste
10	Chemical waste	Chemical used in production of biologicals or disinfection

XIV. HEALTH PLANNING

Chaddah committee:

- NMEP with general health services and Basic health worker per 10,000 population (for malaria vigilance, collection of vital statistics and family planning)

Kartar Singh committee:

- MPHW under Health and family planning (ANMs to be replaced by 'Female Health Workers' and Basic health workers, Malaria surveillance workers, vaccinators, health education assistants to be replaced by 'Male Health Workers')

Bhore committee

- Health survey and development committee
- PHC/primary health centre concept (1 PHC per 40,000 population, 30 beds, 3 subcenters and 2 medical officers)
- 3 months training in PSM (prepare social physicians)

XV. EPIDEMIOLOGY

TYPES OF STUDIES

Case control study/Retrospective study:

- Suitable for: Rare diseases
- Backward looking study
- Effect to cause study
- Disease to risk factor study
- Outcome to cause study
- Rapid
- Easy
- Inexpensive
- No risk to subjects
- Multiple exposures can be checked
- No loss of follow-up
- Requires few subjects
- Cannot measure incidence
- Recall bias is a problem
- Case and control selection troublesome
- Yields: Odd's ratio

Cohort study/Prospective study:

- Reserved for testing of precisely formulated hypothesis
- Best way to identify incidence, natural history of a disease and can be used to examine multiple outcomes after a single exposure
- Forward looking study
- Cause to effect study
- Risk factor to disease study
- Exposure to outcome study
- Follow-up study
- Can examine rare exposures
- Can establish population based incidence
- Time-to-event analysis is possible
- Decreased selection and information bias
- Sampling and observer bias
- Loss to follow-up, migration or non-response bias
- Not suitable for conditions with long latency
- Not suitable for rare diseases
- Lengthy and expensive study
- Yields:
  - o Attributable risk
  - o Relative risk
  - o Incidence

Blind study:

- In single blind study, patient is not aware whether he is in the control or study group
- Double blind study:
  - o Patient does not know which treatment they are receiving
  - o Investigator/doctor does not know which treatment they are giving
- In triple blinding, along with patient and doctor, the person analyzing the data is also unaware/blind

Tip of iceberg phenomenon:

- Bottom of iceberg: Subclinical cases of the disease
- Water-line: Differentiation between apparent and in apparent disease
- Submerged part: Undiagnosed cases in community (latent, presymptomatic cases)
- Floating tip: Clinical cases

Tools of measurement in epidemiology

- Number of new cases occurring during a specified time in a defined population, initially free of disease: Incidence
- Incidence = Prevalence/average duration of the disease
- All cases counted on a single survey or examination of a group: Prevalence

- Occurrence of more cases of a disease than expected in a given area over a particular period of time: Epidemic
- Constant presence of a disease in a defined geographical area: Endemic
- Disease affecting a large geographical area such as part of a nation, continent or world: Pandemic
- Number of infant deaths per thousand live births: Infant Mortality Rate
- Number of maternal deaths per lakh live births: Maternal Mortality Rate
- Number of exposed person's developing the disease within the range of the incubation period following exposure to primary cause: Secondary attack rate
- Time interval between receipt of infection and maximal infectivity: Generation time
- Period between diagnosis by early detection/screening and diagnosis by other (routine) means: Lead time
- Gap between onset of primary case (1st case introduced) and secondary case (develops from primary case): Serial interval
- Number of deaths per 100 cases: Case fatality rate

Screening:

- True positive (sensitivity):
  - o A positive result in the presence of the disease
  - o Ability of screening test to identify correctly all those who have the disease
- True negative (Specificity):
  - o A negative test, in the absence of the disease
  - o Ability of screening test to identify correctly all those who do not have the disease
- Negative predictive value: Ability of a screening test to identify correctly all those who do not have the disease, out of all those who test negative on a screening test
- Positive predictive value: Ability of a screening test to identify correctly all those who have the disease, out of all those who test positive on a screening test

Disease:

- Control: Disease agent is allowed to persist in the community at a level where it ceases to be a public health problem
- Eradication: Termination of all transmission of infection by extermination of the infectious agent
- Elimination: Intermediate goal between disease control and disease elimination

Surveillance:

- The continuous scrutiny of the risk factors that determine the occurrence and distribution of the disease
- Sentinel surveillance: A method for identifying the missing cases and thereby supplementing the notified cases

XVI. CONCEPTS OF HEALTH

Levels of prevention:

- Defluoridation of water/provision of safe water and housing: Primary prevention
- Pap smear: Secondary prevention
- Salt restriction in non-communicable disease: Primordial prevention
- Cessation of smoking: Primordial prevention
- Immunization: Primary prevention
- IOL implantation (treatment) in cataract surgery: Secondary prevention
- Physiotherapy in a case with poliomyelitis: Tertiary prevention

Primordial prevention:

- Prevention of the emergence of the risk factors: Primordial prevention
- Best applied for chronic diseases, coronary artery disease, hypertension (non-communicable)
- Avoidance of smoking and fatty diet
- Exercise to avoid risk of CHD/HTN
- Source reduction in malaria

Primary prevention:

- Action taken prior to onset of disease (health promotion and specific protection-immunization, chemoprophylaxis): Primary prevention
- Best applied for Vaccine preventable diseases
- The action is taken prior to onset of disease (risk factor present)
- Mode of intervention:
  - o Health promotion
  - o Specific protection
- Health promotion:
  - o Health education

- o Lifestyle and behavioural change
- o Nutritional intervention (food fortification)
- o Environmental (safe water and housing)
- Specific protection:
  - o Immunization against VPDs
  - o Vitamin A prophylaxis
  - o Contraception for STDs
  - o Chemoprophylaxis
  - o Protection against occupational hazards, accidents, carcinogens and allergens
  - o Bed nets
  - o Quarantine

Secondary prevention:

- Action halting the progress of disease at early stage (early diagnosis and treatment): Secondary prevention
- Best applied for TB, leprosy, STDs
- Screening test and case finding (pap smear for Ca cervix)
- Treatment of TB, leprosy and STDs
- Its purpose is to cure disease, slow its progression or reduce its impact on individuals or communities

Tertiary prevention:

- Disability limitation and Rehabilitation: Tertiary prevention
- Best applied for polio
- Tertiary prevention strategies involve both therapeutic and rehabilitative measures once disease is firmly established

Must know terms:

- Provision of free medical services to people at GOVERNMENT expenses: State medicine
- Provision of medical services and professional education by STATE, but the programme is operated and regulated by PROFESSIONAL GROUPS rather than government: Socialized medicine
- Any loss/abnormality of psychological, physiologic or anatomical structure or function (e.g., loss of foot, defective vision): Impairment
- Because of impairment, affected person may be unable to carry out certain activities, which may be considered normal for his age, sex (cannot walk): Disability

Indices:

- Infant mortality rate, Life expectancy at ONE year, Literacy rate:
  - o Physical Quality of Life Index/PQLI
  - o Ranges from 0-100
- Expectation of life free of disability: Sullivan's index
- Burden of disease and effectiveness of interventions/Years of life lost to premature death:
  - o Disability Adjusted Life Year/DALY
  - o Highest DALY is for psychiatric disorders (Schizophrenia, unipolar/bipolar disorders)
- Education, Occupation, Income: Kuppuswamy's index

XVII. DEMOGRAPHY AND HEALTH

Demographic cycle:

Crude death rate	Crude birth rate	Phase	Stage
High	High	High stationary	I
Starts declining	High	Early expanding	II
Continue declining	Starts declining	Late expanding	III
Low	Low	Low stationary	IV
High	Low	Declining	V

Other indicators:

- Crude death rate: Total number of deaths in a year/1000 MYP (mid-year population)
- Crude birth rate: Total number of live birth in a year/1000 MYP
- Dependents age group: Above 65 years and below 15 years

XVIII. PSM IN OBSTETRICS AND PEDIATRICS

Fertility indicators:

- Net reproduction rate: Number of daughters a newborn girl will bear during her entire life time assuming fixed age specific fertility and mortality rates

- Gross reproduction rate: Number of daughters a newborn girl will bear during her entire life time if she experiences the current fertility throughout her reproductive age group assuming no mortality
- Total fertility rate: Average number of children a woman would bear in her reproductive age group (child-bearing age)
- General fertility rate: Number of live births per thousand women in the reproductive age group (15 to 45 years)

Intelligence quotient/IQ:

- Calculated as: Mental age × 100/Chronological age
- 0 - 25: Idiot
- 25 - 50: Imbecile
- 50 – 70: Moron
- 70 – 80: Borderline
- 80 – 90: Low normal
- 90 – 110: Normal
- 110 – 120: Superior
- 120 – 140: Very superior
- Above 140: Near Genius

Mental retardation:

- Mild: IQ of 50 – 70
- Moderate: IQ of 35 – 50
- Severe: IQ of 20 – 35
- Profound: IQ of less than 20

5 CHAPTER
Mental Health Nursing

I. GENERAL PSYCHIATRY

Terms and scientists:

- Classical conditioning: Pavlov
- Schizophrenia: Bleuler
- Ambivalence: Bleuler
- Father of attachment theory: John Bowlby
- Adolescent turmoil (stages of life): Erikson
- Catatonia: Kahlbalum

Delusion:

- Disorder of: Disorder of thought (content)
- Defined as: False unshaken belief not amenable to reasoning

Hallucination:

- Disorder of: Disorder of perception
- Definition: Perception in the absence of external stimuli
- Under control of observer: No

Illusion:

- Misinterpretation of external stimuli

II. DELIRIUM

Delirium:

- Most common organic mental disorder seen in clinical practice
- 5-15% patients in medical and surgical inpatient units are estimated to develop delirium at some time in their lives
- % is higher in postoperative patients
- Perceptual disturbances (illusions, misinterpretations and hallucinations)
- Disturbance of sleep-wake cycle (insomnia at night with daytime drowsiness)
- Diurnal variation is marked, usually with worsening of symptoms in the evening and night (sun downing)
- Carphologia/floccillation (picking movements at cover-sheets and clothes)
- Also known as: Acute confusional state

For better preparation and success in AIIMS-NORCET Exam, download **'drkamalkvgroup'** mobile app from Google Playstore.

WhatsApp: +91 84 7000 4333

III. DEMENTIA

Dementia:

- Judgment: Impaired

- Personality changes: Personality alteration (personality deterioration with lack of personal care)
- Consciousness: No disturbance of consciousness

Causes of reversible dementia:

- Hypothyroidism (prompt treatment can reverse the dementing process and lead to complete recovery if the treatment is started within two years of the onset of dementia)
- Hypoparathyroidism
- Hyperparathyroidism etc.

Causes of irreversible dementia:

- Alzheimer's dementia (Most common cause)
- Multi-infarct dementia etc.

Alzheimer's dementia

- Type:
  - o Cortical (NOT subcortical) dementia
  - o Subcortical dementia includes Huntington's chorea, Parkinson's disease, Wilson's disease
- Course: Progressive
- Management:
  - o Donepezil
  - o Rivastigmine
  - o Galantamine

IV. CHILDHOOD PSYCHIATRY

Autism

- Difficulty in: Concentration and communication
- Milestone: Delayed speech and language development
- Clinical features:
  - o Problems in forming social relationships in early childhood
  - o Stereotyped movements
  - o Poor speech
  - o Lack of social interaction

Asperger's syndrome:

- Variant of autism, but WITHOUT any delay in language or cognitive development
- Better prognosis

Attention deficit hyperactivity disorder

- Clinical feature:
  - o Easy distractibility/poor attention span
  - o Impulsivity
- Management:
  - o Methylphenidate
  - o Atomoxetine

For better preparation and success in AIIMS-NORCET Exam, download **'drkamalkvgroup'** mobile app from Google Playstore.

WhatsApp: +91 84 7000 4333

V. SCHIZOPHRENIA

1st rank symptoms of schizophrenia/SFRS:

- Passivity phenomenon
  - o 'Made' feelings/impulses/acts
  - o Somatic passivity
- Hallucination
  - o 3rd person
  - o Voices commenting on one's action
- Delusional perception (thought echo)
- Thought alienation phenomenon:
  - o Thought insertion
  - o Thought withdrawl
  - o Thought broadcasting/diffusion

Bleuler's criterion for schizophrenia (4A's):

- Association disturbance (thought disorder)
- Affect disturbance (anhedonia)
- Autism (withdrawl into self)
- Ambivalence
  - o Marked inability to decide for or against
  - o Double mindedness/confusion

Other important points:

- 1st symptom to go with treatment: Auditory hallucination
- Amphetamines causes: Paranoid schizophrenia
- Late onset schizophrenia comes after the age of: More than 40 years

Good prognostic factor:

- Acute/abrupt in onset
- Late onset type
- Presence of precipitants/stressors
- Depression

VI. MOOD DISORDERS

Depression:

- Most common psychiatric disorder in India:
  - o Generalized anxiety disorder
  - o Depression
- Neurotransmitter involved in depression:
  - o Decreased Serotonin
  - o Decreased Norepinephrine
- Most common cause of suicide: Depression
- Nihilistic ideas are seen in: Depression

Mania:

- Inflated self esteem
- Grandiosity
- Talkativeness
- Flight of ideas
- Distractibility

VII. DRUGS AND PROCEDURES IN PSYCHIATRY

Naltrexone:

- Used in opioid dependency
  - o For rapid detoxification and maintenance therapy
  - o To prevent relapse
- Used to reduce craving and prevent relapse in heavy alcohol drinking (alcohol dependence)

Lithium:

- Therapeutic level: 0.8-1.2 mmol/L
- Prophylactic maintenance level: 0.5-0.8
- Toxicity starts at: >2.0 mEq/L
- Organ NOT affected in toxicity: Liver
- Most common symptoms of toxicity of lithium:
  - o Fine Tremors
  - o Renal failure on long-term therapy
- C/I in: Pregnancy (causes CVS defects)
- Agent of choice for prophylaxis in mania: Lithium (mood stabilizer)

Drug causing depression:

- Steroids (Most common)
- OCP
- Bromocriptine

Electroconvulsive therapy/ECT:

- Indications:
  - o Major severe depression (associated with suicidal risk)
  - o Severe psychosis (schizophrenia/mania) associated with suicidal risk and no response to antipsychotics
  - o Severe functional catatonia etc.
- Absolute C/I for ECT: Raised ICT
- Most common side effect of modified ECT is: Retrograde amnesia (antegrade amnesia also occurs but with decreased frequency)
- Effect of ECT on intraocular tension: Decrease

VIII. ALCOHOL

Alcoholism:

- Korsakoff's syndrome presents as:
  - o Profound – persistent anterograde amnesia
  - o Gross memory disturbances
  - o Confabulation
- Questionnaire used:
  - o C: Cut down (amount)
  - o A: Annoyed by people
  - o G: Guilt of drinking
  - o E: Early morning/eye opener drink

Alcohol withdrawal:

- Most common syndrome of Alcohol withdrawal: Hangover next morning
- Most severe syndrome of Alcohol withdrawal: Delirium tremens
- Delirium tremens is characterized by:
  - o Disorientation
  - o Anxiety
  - o Perceptual defect
- Drug used for managing delirium tremens: Chlordiazepoxide

IX. MISCELLANOUS TOPICS

Somatization disorder:

- Patient presents with multiple physical complaints (referable to different organ systems) in the absence of any physical disorder
- Symptoms are recurrent and chronic (at least 2 years duration is needed for diagnosis)
- Symptoms:
  - o Gastrointestinal (abdominal pain, belching, nausea, vomiting)
  - o Abnormal skin sensations (numbness, soreness)
  - o Sexual and menstrual complaints
- Frequent change of treating physicians
- Persistent refusal to accept the advice or reassurance

Hypochondriasis:

- Essential feature:
  - o Belief of serious medical illness that persists despite reassurance and appropriate medical evaluation
  - o Abnormal pre-occupation
  - o Normal body functions

Impulse control disorders

- Dipsomania: Irresistible desire for alcohol drinks
- Trichotillomania: Need to pull out hair
- Pyromania: Irresistible desire to set things on fire
- Kleptomania: Irresistible desire to steal articles

Phobic disorders:

- Marked and persistent fear of objects/situations, exposure to which results in immediate anxiety reaction
- Agoraphobia (Most common type):
  - o Old: Fear of open spaces
  - o Now: Places from where there is no easy escape to safe place
- Claustrophobia: Fear of closed spaces
- Management of phobia:
  - o Cognitive behavioural therapy/systemic desensitization (best)
  - o Alprazolam
  - o SSRI (paroxetine)

Sleep

- Alpha waves are seen in: Eyes closed, mind wandering
- Night terrors are seen in: NREM sleep
- Sleep walking/somnabulism is seen in: NREM sleep (stage 3/4)
- Sleep terror/Pavor nocturnus is seen in:
  - o NREM sleep (stage 3/4)
  - o Treated by diazepam

Obsessive compulsive disorder:

- Neurotransmitter implicated: Serotonin
- Features of OCD:
- Obsessive thoughts and compulsive behaviors that impair everyday functioning
  - o Repetitive thoughts/images
  - o Shows perfectionism

- Management of OCD:
  - Fluoxetine (DOC)
  - Fluoxamine
  - Exposure and response prevention

Mental health and Mental retardation

- Normal IQ: 90-110
- IQ is calculated as: (Mental age/chronological age) × 100
- Mental ill health is usually due to: Social maladjustment
- Chromosomal abnormality causing MR:
  - Down syndrome (Most common)
  - Fragile X syndrome (2nd Most common)
- Mild MR: 50-70

6 CHAPTER

Pharmacology

I. GENERAL PHARMACOLOGY

Pharmacokinetics:

- It is the study of "what the body does to a drug"
- It is a quantitative study of drug movement in through and out of the body
- This refers to movement of the drug in and alteration of the drug by the body. It includes:
    - o Absorption
    - o Distribution
    - o Binding/localization/storage
    - o Biotransformation
    - o Excretion of the drug

Therapeutic window phenomenon:

- Optimal effect is exerted only over a narrow range of plasma drug concentration
- Between minimal therapeutic effect and the dose which produces maximal acceptable adverse effect
- E.g. TCA, clonidine, glipizide

Therapeutic index:

- Toxic dose/Therapeutic dose
- Median lethal dose/Median effective dose
- LD_{50}/ED_{50}

Drug efficacy:

- Maximal effect that a drug may elicit
- Upper limit of DRC (dose-response curve)
- Morphine produces a degree of analgesia NOT obtainable with any dose of aspirin – Morphine is more efficacious than aspirin

Drug potency:

- Amount of drug required to produce a certain response
- Factor in choosing the dose of a drug
- Position of DRC on the dose axis
- More rightward = Lower potency
- 10 mg of morphine = 100 mg of pethidine as analgesic. Morphine is 10 times more potent than pethidine

BA:

- Bioavailability/BA by intravenous route is: 100%
- Fraction of drug that reaches the systemic circulation in the unchanged form

Pro-drugs:

- Enalapril → Enalaprilat
- Levodopa → Dopamine
- Prednisone → Prednisolone
- Sulfasalazine → 5-ASA

First order reaction:

- Constant FRACTION of drug is eliminated
- CL remains constant
- Rate of elimination is directly DEPENDENT on plasma concentration
- $t_{1/2}$ is constant

Zero order reaction/Capacity limited elimination/Michaelis-Menten elimination:

- Constant AMOUNT is excreted
- Clearance/CL decreases with increase in concentration
- Rate of elimination INDEPENDENT of plasma concentration
- Variable $t_{1/2}$
- E.g., Ethyl alcohol

First order → zero order kinetics:

- Higher doses
- Plasma concentration increases disproportionately with increase in dose
- E.g., Phenytoin, Warfarin

Drug absorption:

- Basic drugs (morphine, quinine) are absorbed from: Proximal intestine (duodenum)
- Acidic drugs (salicylates, barbiturates) are predominantly unionized in the acid gastric juice and are absorbed from stomach

Microsomal enzymes:

- Located on SER
- Liver, kidney, intestinal mucosa and lungs
- Mono-oxygenase, cytochrome-P450 etc.
- Catalyze most of the oxidations, reductions, hydrolysis and glucuronide conjugation

Extra-pyramidal side-effects:

- Drugs causing extrapyramidal side effects:
  - Haloperidol
  - Levodopa
- Parkinsonism:
  - Acute muscular dystonia: Bizarre muscle spasms
  - Akathisia: Restlessness
  - Malignant Neuroleptic syndrome: Rigidity, hyperthermia
  - Tardive dyskinesia: Purposeless involuntary facial and limb movements

FIRST PASS METABOLISM

First pass/presystemic metabolism:

- Metabolism of a drug during its passage from the site of absorption into systemic circulation
- Orally absorbed drugs → drug metabolizing enzymes in the intestinal wall and liver (through portal vein)
- Rectal route

FPM is avoided by administering the drug through:

- Sublingual
- Transdermal
- Parenteral routes

Drugs with HIGH first pass metabolism/FPM:

- High oral dose:
  - Beta blockers (propranolol)
  - Salbutamol
- Not given orally:
  - Lignocaine
  - Isoprenaline

CLINICAL TRIALS

Clinical trial:

- It is a prospective ethically designed investigation in human subjects to objectively discover/verify/compare the results of two or more therapeutic measures (drugs)

Phase I:

- Human pharmacology and safety
- Administration carried out by highly qualified clinical pharmacologists/physician
- In a setting where all vital functions are monitored
- Emergency resuscitative facilities are available
- 20-80 Subjects (healthy mostly)
- Starting with the lowest estimated dose
- Emphasis is on safety, tolerability, and to detect any potentially dangerous effects on vital functions

Phase II:

- Therapeutic exploration and dose ranging
- Conducted by physician who are trained as clinical investigators
- 100-500 patients selected
- Primary aim is to establishment of therapeutic efficacy, dose range and ceiling effect in controlled setting
- Drug may be dropped if desired level of clinical efficacy is NOT obtained

Phase III:

- Therapeutic confirming/Comparison
- Randomized double blind comparative trials
- 500-3000 patients
- Several physicians (specialist in treating the target disease)
- Aim is to establish the value of the drug in relation to existing therapy
- A 'NDA' is submitted to the licensing authority for permission

Phase IV:

- Post marketing surveillance/studies
- After the drug has been marketed for general use
- Practising physicians are identified through whom
- Data is collected on structured proforma
- About efficacy, acceptability and adverse effects of the drug
- Patient number is much larger
- Idiosyncratic/uncommon adverse effects or those which occurs on long-term use and unsuspected drug interactions are detected

Summary:

- I: Human safety
- II: Drug efficacy
- III: Comparison
- IV: Side effects/interactions

Phase 0/Microdosing study:

- Strategy developed to reduce down the cost and time of the drug development process
- Very low doses (1/100th of the estimated human dose are adminstered to healthy volunteers)

II. DRUGS ACTING ON AUTONOMIC NERVOUS SYSTEM

Atropine:

- Uses of atropine (more potent action on heart, bronchial muscles and intestines)
- Organophosphate poisoning
- Early Mushroom/Inocybe poisoning
- Treating bradyarrhythmias and partial heart block (selected cases)
- Pre-anaesthetic medications (reduces secretions)
- Treatment of iritis, iridocyclitis, choroiditis, keratitis and corneal ulcer

ADRENERGIC SYSTEM

Functions of alpha 1 receptors:

- Genitourinary smooth muscle contraction
- Vasoconstriction
- Gland – secretion
- Gut – relaxation
- Alpha1 agonist:
  - o Phenylephrine
  - o Methoxamine
- Alpha1 blockers:
  - o Prazosin
  - o Tamsulosin

Functions of alpha 2 receptors:

- Inhibition of transmitter release
- Vasoconstriction
- Decreased central sympathetic flow
- Alpha 2 agonist:
  - o Decreased central sympathetic flow
  - o Clonidine
  - o Methyldopa
- Alpha 2 blockers:
  - o Yohimbine
  - o Mirtazapine (antidepressant)
  - o Rauwolscine

Beta1 agonist:

- Isoproterenol (beta1 = beta2)
- Dobutamine (beta1 > beta2)
- Beta1 blocker:
  - o Acebutolol
  - o Atenolol
  - o Betaxolol

- o Bisoprolol
- o Esmolol
- o Metoprolol

Beta2 agonist:

- Salbutamol
- Salmeterol
- Terbutaline
- Ritodrine

Beta1 and Beta2 blocker:

- Dilevelol
- Labetalol
- Carvedilol (alpha1, beta1, beta2 blocker)

III. AUTACOIDS

SEROTONIN RECEPTORS

5HT 1A agonist:

- 5-HT 1A: Present in hippocampus
- Buspirone (antianxiety)

5HT 1B agonist:

- Constricts cranial blood vessels
- Sumitriptan (migraine)

5HT 4 agonist:

- Mediates intestinal secretion
- Augmentation of peristalsis
- Cisapride
- Renzapride (increases gastric motility)

5HT 2A antagonist:

- Post-junctional receptor mediating direct actions of 5-HT like vascular and visceral smooth muscle contraction, platelet aggregation, neuronal activation in brain
- Cyproheptadine
- Ketanserin

5HT 2A/2C antagonist:

- Clozapine

5HT 3 antagonist:

- Depolarizes neurons by gating cation channels; elicits reflex effects of 5-HT: emesis, gut peristalsis, bradycardia
- Ondansetron

PROSTAGLANDIN

PGE1:

- Misoprostol: Treatment of NSAID induced ulcer
- Alprostadil:
  - o Maintains ductus arteriosus
  - o Impotence

PGE2:

- Dinoprostone: Induction/augmentation of labor, midterm abortion

PGF 2 alpha:

- Latanoprost/Travopost/Bimatoprost: Treatment of glaucoma (lowers intraocular tension by enhancing uveo-oscleral and trabecular outflow)
- Latanoprost are now the first line drugs from wide angle glaucoma

PGI2:

- Epoprostenol: Prevent platelet aggregation and damage during hemodialysis

IV. DRUGS RELATED TO ENDOCRINE SYSTEM

CORTICOIDS

Aldosterone:

- Maximum mineralocorticoid activity is shown by: Aldosterone
- The principal mineralocorticoid action is enhancement of sodium reabsorption in the distal convoluted tubule in kidney.
- There is associated increase in K^+ and H^+ excretion

Glucocorticoid:

- Maximum glucocorticoid activity is shown by:
  - o Dexamethasone
  - o Betamethasone (Zero mineralocorticoid)
- Glucorticoid inhibit glucose utilization by peripheral tissues
- This along with increased glucose release from liver results in hyperglycemia, resistance to insulin and a diabetes-like state
- They also cause protein breakdown and amino acid mobilization from peripheral tissues
- This is responsible for side effects like muscle wasting, lympholysis, loss of osteoid from bone and thinning of skin
- Subcutaneous tissue over extremities loses fat which is deposited over face, neck and shoulder producing 'moon face', 'fish mouth' and 'buffalo hump'
- Glucocorticoids inhibit intestinal absorption and enhance renal excretion of calcium
- Loss of osteoid indirectly results in loss of calcium from bone
- Secretion of gastric acid and pepsin is increased – may aggravate peptic ulcer
- Irrespective of the type of injury or insult, the attending inflammatory response is suppressed by glucorticoids
- This is the basis of most of their clinical uses
- Glucocorticoids impair immunological competence
- They suppress all types of hypersensitization and allergic phenomena

Clomiphene:

- Anti-estrogen drug is: Clomiphene
- It binds to both estrogen receptors (ER-alpha and ER-beta) and acts as pure estrogen antagonist in all human tissues
- It induces Gn secretion in women by blocking estrogenic feedback inhibition of pituitary
- The amount of LH/FSH released at each secretory pulse is increased. In response, the ovaries enlarge and ovulation occurs

Tamoxifen:

- MOA of tamoxifen: Oral Selective Estrogen Receptor Modulator (SERM). It has a complex action
- Acts as potent estrogen antagonist in breast carcinoma cells, blood vessels and at some peripheral sites, but as partial agonist in uterus, bone, liver and pituitary.

V. ANTIDIABETIC DRUG

Biguanides:

- Effect of metformin (biguanide) on glucose metabolism:
  - o Overcome insulin resistance
  - o Enhances insulin mediated glucose uptake and disposal in skeletal muscle and fat (Increased glycolysis)
  - o Decreased hepatic gluconeogensis and glucose output from liver
- Special feature of metformin:
  - o It does not cause weight gain (so particularly used in obesity; obesity is NOT a contraindication)
  - o Does NOT cause hypoglycemia (non-hypoglycemic)
- Feared complication of metformin: Lactic acidosis (More with phenformin and banned in India since 2003 for this particular side effect)
- Metformin is C/I in:
  - o Hypotensive states
  - o Heart failure
  - o Severe respiratory
  - o Hepatic diseases
  - o Renal disease
  - o In alcoholics
  - o Because of increased risk of lactic acidosis in all the above conditions

Starch Inhibitor:

- MOA of Acarbose and Miglitol (alpha glucosidase/starch inhibitor):
  - o Decreases progression of impaired glucose tolerance to overt disease Slows down and decrease digestion and absorption of polysaccharides and sucrose
- Special feature of Acarbose and Miglitol: They are mild anti-hyperglycaemics

Pioglitazone:

- Effect of Pioglitazone (thiazolidine-diones) is: Acts by binding to PPAR-gamma (peroxisome proliferator activator receptors-gamma)
- Increases insulin sensitivity of tissues (reverse insulin resistance)

INSULIN

Insulin:

- $t_{1/2}$ of Insulin: 5 minutes

- Effect of Insulin on potassium: Promotes entry of potassium into the cell
- Difference between human and pork insulin: 1 amino acid

INSULIN PREPARATIONS

Rapid acting insulin:

- Insulin aspart
- Lispro insulin
- Insulin glusuline

Long acting insulin:

- Insulin glargine
- Insulin detemir

V. DRUGS ACTING ON CARDIOVASCULAR SYSTEM

ANTIHYPERTENSIVES

ACE Inhibitors:

- ACE inhibitors causes cough because of: Bradykinin
- C/I of ACE inhibitors:
  - o Bilateral renal artery stenosis (due to dilatation of efferent arterioles and fall in glomerular filtration pressure)
  - o Pregnancy (hypoplasia of organs)
  - o Phaeochromocytoma
- Act by blocking conversion of angiotensin I to angiotensin II, decreases vasopressor activity of angiotensin II and aldosterone secretion by increasing bradykinin (causes a fall in total peripheral resistance)
- Side effects inlcude angioedema, dry cough, hyperkalemia, taste alteration, azotemia etc.
- Members include captopril, enalapril, lisinopril

DRUGS USED IN HEART FAILURE

Digoxin:

- Therapeutic level of digoxin: 0.5 to 1.4 ng/ml
- Toxic level of digoxin: More than 2 ng/ml
- MOA of digoxin:
  - o Inhibit Na^+/K^+ ATPase
  - o Increases ventricular contractile force
- Route of excretion of digoxin: Kidneys
- C/I of digoxin: HOCM
- Digoxin (electrolyte abnormality) toxicity consists of:
  - o Hypokalemia (classical finding)
  - o Hypomagnesemia

Nitrates:

- Effects of nitrates on CVS physiology:
  - o Decreases preload and afterload
  - o Decreases myocardial oxygen consumption
- S/E of nitrates:
  - o Hypotension
  - o Reflex tachycardia
- Long acting nitrates are NOT used chronically as: Tolerance develops (due to –SH group)

VI. DRUGS ACTING ON NERVOUS SYSTEM

ANTIDEPRESSANTS

TCA:

- Amitryptyline
- Clomipramine

Tetracyclic antidepressants (second generation):

- Maprotiline

SSRI's:

- Fluoxetine

ANTI-EPILEPTICS

Side effect (S/E) of phenytoin:

- Gum hyperplasia

- Hydantoin syndrome
- Cerebellar atrophy
- Megaloblastic anemia
- Pseudo-Lymphoma

VII. DRUGS ACTING ON RESPIRATORY SYSTEM

ANTI-ASTHMATICS

Theophylline (Methylxanthine):

- Theophylline metabolizing enzymes are saturable, $t^{1/2}$ is prolonged with higher doses as kinetics changes from first to zero order
- Plasma concentrations, therefore increase disproportionately with dose
- It has a narrow margin of safety

Uses of theophylline:

- Bronchial asthma and COPD (Use in asthma has declined because of narrow margin of safety and limited efficacy)
- It is more useful in COPD
- Apnoea in premature infant

MOA of theophylline and doxophylline:

- Inhibits phosphodiesterase 4 (PDE4)
  - o Theophylline is a subtype nonselective and weak PDE inhibitor, but PDE4 inhibition is mainly responsible for bronchodilatation
- Release of Ca^{2+} from sarcoplasmic reticulum, especially in skeletal muscle and cardiac muscle
- Blockade of adenosine receptors

Sodium cromoglycate:

- Not absorbed orally
- Administered as an aerosol through metered dose inhaler
- MOA of sodium chromoglycate/Cromolyn sodium (used for prophylaxis):
  - o Inhibitor of mast cell degranulation (as well as other inflammatory cells) by trigger stimuli
  - o Release of mediators of asthma like histamine, leukotrienes, PAF interleukins, etc, is restricted

Uses of Cromolyn sodium:

- Bronchial asthma (long-term prophylactic in mild-moderate asthma)
- Allergic rhinitis and allergic conjunctivitis

Montelukast:

- MOA of Montelukast:
  - o Leukotriene receptor antagonist/LTRA
  - o It competitively antagonize $cysLT_1$ receptor mediated bronchoconstriction, airway mucus secretion, increased vascular permeability and recruitment of eosinophils

Uses of monteleukast:

- Used in maintenance therapy of asthma (prophylactic therapy for mild-moderate asthma as alternatives to inhaled glucocorticoids)
- Modestly effective in asprin-induced asthma and exercise induced asthma

Monteleukast is NOT useful in:

- Acute attacks of asthma (they are not to be used for terminating asthma episodes)

Steroids in asthma:

- They are not bronchodilators
- They benefit by reducing bronchial hyperactivity, mucosal edema and suppressing inflammatory response to AG : AB (antigen : antibody) reaction
- Systemic steroid therapy is resorted to in asthma in severe chronic asthma (not controlled by bronchodilators and inhaled steroids), status asthmaticus/acute asthma exacerbation and COPD
- S/E of inhaled steroids (Beclomethasone dipropionate, Budesonide and Fluticasone):
  - o Oropharyngeal candidiasis, hoarseness of voice, dysphonia, sore throat
  - o These can be minimized by the use of a spacer, gargling after every dose (to wash off the drug deposited on oral and pharyngeal mucosa) and prevented as well as treated by topical nystatin/clotrimazole
- S/E of topical steroids: Glaucoma
- S/E of parenteral steroids: Posterior subcapsular cataract

VIII. ANTI-BACTERIAL DRUGS

Trimethorpim/TMP:

- MOA of trimethoprim: Inhibit nucleotide synthesis of tetrahydrofolate by inhibiting DHFRase (Dihydrofolate Reductase)
- Related to the antimalarial drug pyrimethamine, which selectively inhibits DHFRase
- TMP is >50,000 times more active against bacterial DHFRase than against the mammalian enzyme. Thus, human folate metabolism is not interfered at antibacterial concentrations of TMP

Cotrimoxazole:

- Individually, both sulfonamide and trimethoprim are bacteriostatic, but the combination becomes cidal against many organisms
- Ratio of sulfamethoxazole/SMO: TMP is 5:1, because TMP enters many tissues, has a large of volume of distribution than SMO and attains lower plasma concentrations
- DOC in p. carinii and nocardiosis: Co-trimoxazole/CTM (pneumocystis jiroveci causes severe pneumonia in neutropenic and AIDS patients; CTM has prophylactic as well as therapeutic value, but high doses are needed)

Fluoroquinolones/FQs:

- Block DNA topoisomerases IV (gram-positive), which nicks and separates daughter DNA strands after DNA replication
- Inhibit bacterial DNA gyrase (gram-negative), which nicks double stranded DNA, introduces negative supercoils and then reseals the nicked ends
- In place of DNA gyrase or topoisomerase IV, the mammalian cell possess an enzyme topoisomerase II (that also removes positive supercoils) which has very low affinity for FQs – hence the low toxicity to host cells

Levofloxacin:

- Oral bioavailability is nearly 100%
- Single dose is sufficient because of slower elimination and higher potency
- Indicated in community acquired pneumonia and exacerbations of chronic bronchitis.
- DOC in legionella: Azithromycin/Levofloxacin

Cephalosporin effective against gram-negative enterobacteriacea (3rd generation):

- Parenteral:
  - o Cefoperazone (anti-pseudomonal activity)
  - o Cefotaxime
  - o Ceftriaxone
  - o Ceftazidime
  - o Ceftizoxime
- Oral:
  - o Cefixime
  - o Cefpodoxime
  - o Cefdinir
  - o Ceftibuten
  - o Ceftamet

Ceftriaxone:

- Longer duration of action (half life: 8 hours), permitting once, or at the most twice daily dosing
- Hypoprothrombinaemia and bleeding are the specific adverse effects
- DOC in gonorrhea: Ceftriaxone (a single dose of 250 mg I/V has proven curative in gonorrhoea)

Imipenem:

- It is inhibited by: Dehydropeptidase I (hence given along with cilastatin)
- Imipenem is an extremely potent and broad-spectrum beta-lactam antibiotic
- Cilastatin has matched pharmacokinetics with imipenem (half-life of both is 1 hour)

Azithromycin:

- Azalide congener of erythromycin
- High activity over respiratory pathogens
- Acid-stability, rapid oral absorption (from empty stomach), larger volume of distribution
- Doesn't affect hepatic CYP3A4 enzyme
- Azithromycin is effective against:
  - o Chlamydia trachomatis (non-specific urethritis and genital infections, LGV, chlamydial pneumonia)
  - o Mycoplasma
  - o Calymmatobacter granulomatosis (donovanosis)
  - o Legionella (Legionnaire's disease)
  - o Chancroid

Tetracycline/TTC:

- Primarily bacteriostatic
- Inhibit protein synthesis by binding to 30S ribosomes

- Subsequent to such binding, attachment of aminoacyl-tRNA to the acceptor (A) site of mRNA-ribosome complex is interfered with
- Most TTC are primarily excreted in urine by glomerular filtration; dose has to be reduced in renal failure; doxycycline is an exception to this
- Demeclocycline antagonizes ADH action and hence tried in inappropriate ADH secretion
- Complication arising due to use of outdated tetracycline/TTC:
    - o Reversible Fanconi's syndrome (caused by degraded products – epitetracycline, anhydrotetracycline and epianhydrotetracycline which damage proximal tubules in kidney)
- S/E of tetracycline:
    - o Teratogenic
    - o Super-infections (TTC cause more marked suppression of the resident flora
        - – Intestinal superinfection by candida albicans is most prominent
        - – Higher doses suppress the flora more completely – greater chance of superinfection so doses on lower side of range should be used whenever possible)
    - o Tooth discoloration (TTC have chelating property)
        - – Calcium-TTC chelate gets deposited in developing teeth and bone
        - – Given from midpregnancy to 5 months of extra-uterine life, the deciduous teeth are affected)
- S/E of doxycycline: Photodermatitis (but highest with Demeclocycline and low with TTC)

Chloramphenicol/CMP:

- Primarily bacteriostatic
- CMP was highly active against Salmonella including S. typhi
- Highly chloramphenicol resistant S. typhi have emerged due to transfer of R factor by conjugation
- It crosses placenta and is secreted in bile and milk
- Primarily conjugated with glucuronic acid in the liver and little is excreted unchanged in urine
- It is most important cause of aplastic anemia, agranulocytosis and thrombocytopenia (bone marrow depression)
- MOA of chloramphenicol: Bind to 50s subunit near the acceptor (A) site and prevents peptide bond formation between the newly attached amino acid and the nascent peptide chain without interfering with the aminoacyl-tRNA attachment to the 30S ribosomes (the step blocked by TTC)

Penicillin-G/PnG:

- Narrow spectrum antibiotic
- Penicillinase is a narrow spectrum beta-lactamase which opens the beta-lactam ring and inactivates PnG
- Use has declined very much due to fear of causing anaphylaxis
- DOC in syphilis: Penicillin G (T. pallidum has not shown any resistance and PnG is the drug of choice)
- DOC in actinomycosis: Penicillin-G (PnG is the drug of choice for rare infections like anthrax, actinomycosis, rat bite fever and those caused by Listeria monocytogenes, Pasteurella multicoda)
- Chemoprophylactic agent for Rheumatic fever: Benzathine penicillin/BPn (low concentrations of penicillin prevent colonization by streptococci that are indirectly responsible for rheumatic fever; BPn 1.2 MU every 4 weeks till 18 years of age or 5 years after an attack, whichever is more)

AMINOGLYCOSIDES

MOA of aminoglycosides/AGS:

- Inhibit translation (transport of the aminoglycoside through the bacterial cell wall and cytoplasmic membrane followed by binding to 30S ribosomes by streptomycin; other AGS bind to additional sites on 50S subunit as well as to 30S-50S interface)
- Bactericidal (this action is concentration dependent; i.e., rate of bacterial cell killing is directly related to the ratio of the peak antibiotic concentration to the MIC value. They also exert a long and concentration dependent 'postantibiotic effect')
- Distributed only extracellularly

S/E of aminoglycosides:

- Teratogenic (fetal ototoxicity)
- Ototoxic (most important dose and duration of treatment related adverse effect)
- Nephrotoxic (provided the drug is promptly discontinued, renal damage caused by aminoglycosides is totally reversible)
- Causes neuromuscular blockade (reduce Ach release from the motor nerve endings; Neomycin and streptomycin have higher propensity whereas tobramycin is least likely to produce this side effect; this can be partially antagonized by I/V injection of a calcium salt) (should not be used in myasthenia gravis)

Streptomycin:

- Obtained from Streptomyces griseus
- Relatively narrow antimicrobial spectrum

- Can cause vestibular disturbances
- Lowest nephrotoxicity among aminoglycosides
- Streptomycin is used in:
  - o Plague (effects rapid cure in 7-12 days; TTC have been more commonly used for mass treatment of suspected cases during an epidemic)
  - o Tularemia (effects cure in 7-10 days)

IX. ANTI-MALARIAL DRUGS

Quinine:

- DOC for cerebral malaria: Quinine
- S/E of quinine:
  - o Cinchonism: Ringing in ears, nausea, vomiting, difficulty in hearing and visual defects
  - o Hemolysis → hemoglobinuria (black water fever)
  - o Hypoglycemia (especially in pregnancy)

Primaquine:

- Primaquine is effective for: Radical cure of plasmodium vivax
- Primaquine is ineffective against: Plasmodium falciparum
- S/E of primaquine: Hemolysis in G6PD deficients

X. ANTI-FUNGAL DRUGS

Amphotericin B:

- Disrupts fungal cell membrane by binding to ergosterol
- The polyenes (AMB) have high affinity for ergosterol present in fungal cell membrane
- They combine with it, get inserted into the membrane and several polyene molecule together orient themselves in such a way as to form a 'micropore'
- MOA of amphotericin B: Forms micropores in fungal cell membrane (it has affinity for ergosterol)
- Used for systemic mycoses and intrathecally for fungal meningitis
- It binds to ergosterol and forms pores in membrane which promote leakage of electrolytes
- Side effects include shake and bake (fever/chills), arrhythmias, I/V phlebitis (amphoterrible), nephrotoxicity
- Toxicity can be reduced by hydration and liposomal preparation
- AMB is given as I/V solution after diluting AMB powder with glucose solution
- Conventional formulation of Amphotericin B/C-AMB intravenously, is given along with: Glucose solution (after test dose)

KCZ:

- Used for candida, blastomyces and histoplasma
- Side effects include liver dysfunction (as it inhibits cytochrome P-450) and gynecomastia
- MOA of ketoconazole: Inhibits fungal lanosterol 14-demethylase, Impairing ergosterol (fungal steroid) synthesis

XI. ANTI-HIV DRUGS

NRTI group:

- They inhibit reverse transcriptase enzyme thus preventing incorporation of viral genome into host DNA
- Members include Zidovudine, Zalcitabine, Lamivudine, Abacavir, Didanosine and Stavudine

Abacavir:

- Belongs to Nucleoside reverse transcriptase inhibitor
- Guanosine analogue

NNRTIs group:

- Same as that of NRTI group
- Members include Nevirapine, Etravirine, Delaviridine and Efavirenz
- Nevirapine and Efavirenz belongs to: Non-nucleoside reverse transcriptase inhibitor

Protease inhibitor group:

- They block protease in progeny virions thus inhibiting assembly of new virus
- Members include Ritonavir, Nelfinavir, Saquinavir, Indinavir, Amprenavir
- Saquinavir and Nelfinavir belongs to: Protease inhibitor

S/E of Zidovudine:

- Myelosuppression
- Megaloblastic anemia (macrocytosis)
- Neutropenia
- Myopathy (skeletal and cardiac)

S/E of didanosine:

- Pancreatitis

- Peripheral neuropathy
- Hyperuricemia
- Seizures etc.

XII. ANTI-TUBERCULAR DRUGS

INH:

- MOA of Isoniazid/INH: Inhibits mycolic acid cell wall synthesis via oxygen-dependent pathways
- Anti-TB drug showing maximum resistance in India: INH
- Special feature about activity of INH:
  - o Bacteriostatic against resting bacilli
  - o Bacteriocidal against rapidly multiplying organism (both intracellularly and extracellularly present organism)
- Treatment of INH related peripheral neuritis:
  - o 100 mg of pyridoxine daily for treatment
  - o 10 mg/day for prophylaxis (orally)
- S/E of INH:
  - o Peripheral neuritis (common in slow acetylator)
  - o Hepatotoxicity (common in elderly and alcoholics; rare in children)
  - o Seizures (neurotoxicity)
  - o Optic neuritis
  - o Hemolysis in G-6-PD deficients
  - o SLE like syndrome

S/E of rifampicin:

- Respiratory syndrome
- Abdominal syndrome
- Flu like syndrome
- Cutaneous syndrome
- Hepatotoxicity
- Orange coloured urine and sweat
- P-450 drug interactions (microsomal enzyme inducer) etc.

Pyrazinamide:

- Special features of pyrazinamide:
  - o Levels in CSF are high (good penetration in CSF)
  - o Bacteriocidal to organism lying within caseous granuloma (acidic pH) and slowly dividing intracellular bacteria
- MOA of pyrazinamide:
  - o Similar to INH (inhibition of mycolic acid cell wall synthesis) but by interacting with a different fatty acid synthase encoding gene (but intracellular action)
  - o More active at pH <6
- Side effects (3H):
  - o Hepatotoxicity (less in Indians)
  - o Hyperuricemia
  - o Hyperglycemia

S/E of ethambutol:

- Retrobulbar optic neuritis
- Color vision disturbance (red-green)
- Never given to children less than 5 years of age as they can't complain about visual problems

XIII. ANTI-LEPROTIC DRUGS

Rifampicin:

- Most rapidly acting drug against leprosy bacillus: Rifampicin
- Most potent drug against leprosy bacillus: Rifampicin

Dapsone:

- DOC for leprosy: Dapsone
- S/E of dapsone: Hemolysis in G6PD deficient

S/E of clofazimine:

- Reddish black discoloration of skin
- Acneform eruptions

XIV. ANTI-PARASITIC DRUGS

MNZ:

- It is bactericidal
- It forms toxic metabolites in the bacterial cell damaging DNA
- Used as antiprotozoal drug (amoebiasis, giardiasis, bacterial vaginosis) and triple therapy for H. pylori
- Can lead to Disulfiram-like reaction, metallic taste
- DOC for dracunculiasis: Metronidazole/MNZ

7 CHAPTER Microbiology & Parasitology

SECTION 1: MICROBIOLOGY

I. GENERAL MICROBIOLOGY

BASICS

Prokaryotes:

- In prokaryotes, nuclear membrane is: Absent
- In prokaryotes, cellular organelles are: Absent
- They do not have organelles except ribsomes (70s)
- They contain single circular molecule of loosely organized DNA lacking a nuclear membrane and mitotic apparatus

Conjugation (horizontal gene transfer):

- Donor is determined by specific conjugate plasmids called fertility plasmids (F+) or sex plasmids
- Multiple drug resistance

Exotoxin and Endotoxin:

- Mostly secreted by gram-positive bacteria: Exotoxin
- Endotoxin is secreted only by gram-negative bacteria (component of cell wall)
- Highly toxic: Exotoxin
- Endotoxin have low toxicity
- Highly antigenic: Exotoxin (induces synthesis of protective antibody in host called antitoxin)
- Endotoxin is poorly antigenic
- Toxoids are used as vaccines: Exotoxin
- No toxoids, so no vaccines from endotoxin

II. BACTERIOLOGY

STAPHYLOCOCCUS AUREUS

Staph aureus:

- Gram +
- Causes folliculitis, bullous impetigo, osteomyelitis, surgical wound infections
- Food poisoning results due to: Preformed enterotoxin
- Incubation period of staph. aureus food poisoning: Less than 6 hours

- Staph. aureus food poisoning is seen after ingestion of: Dairy products

STREPTOCOCCI

Disease caused by Streptococcus pyogenes (GABHS):

- Pharyngitis/sore throat
- Scarlet fever
- Impetigo
- Erysipelas
- Cellulitis
- Toxic Shock Syndrome (2nd Most common)

PNEUMOCOCCUS

Pneumococcus:

- Alpha hemolytic
- Bile soluble, Optochin sensitive
- Quellung reaction (capsular polysaccharide antigen)
- C-reactive protein (precipitates C-carbohydrate antigen)
- Most common cause of lobar pneumonia and pyogenic meningitis
- Most virulent type of pneumococcus: Type C
- Appearance of colonies: Draughtsman colonies
- Gross appearance of pneumococcus: Lanceolate, Flame shaped diplococcus

NEISSERIA

Condition caused by N. gonorrhoeae:

- Ophthalmia neonatorum (babies born to infected mother)
- Male: Urethritis (does not involve testis)
- Female: Cervicitis
- Complications:
  - o Deep gonococcal infections
  - o Endocarditis (rarely)
  - o Commonly purulent arthritis

N. meningitidis:

- Capsulated
- Lens shaped, half moon shaped (adjacent surfaces flat)
- Ferments glucose and maltose
- Waterhouse-Friderichsen syndrome (fulminant meningococcemia)
- Thayer-Martin media (culture media)

CORYNEBACTERIUM DIPHTHERIAE

C. diphtheriae:

- Club-shaped, irregularly stained gram-positive pleomorphic rod
- Chinese letter/cuneiform arrangement (V-L shaped in smear)

B. ANTHRACIS

B. anthracis:

- Gram +ve, large rectangular rods arranged in chains, non-motile and capsulated, non-bulging oval spores
- It was the first pathogenic bacterium seen under microscope
- Anthrax vaccine was the 1st live attenuated bacterial vaccine prepared

CLOSTRIDIA

C. difficile:

- Obligate anaerobic, gram-positive, spore forming bacillus
- It was so named due to unusual difficulties involved in the isolation of C. difficile
- Clostridium difficile causes:
  - o Pseudomembranous colitis (particularly after antibiotic therapy)
  - o Prolonged antimicorbial use results in disruption of the normal colonic flora, which enhances the susceptibility to C. difficile infection
  - o Ceftriaxone, clindamycin, ampicillin and ciprofloxacin are implicated

C. perfringens/C. welchii:

- Commensal in the large intestine of human beings
- Capsulated, non-motile, gram-positive bacillus
- Clostridium perfringens causes:
  - o Gas gangrene/myonecrosis
  - o Necrotizing enterocolitis
  - o Food poisoning
  - o Enteritis necroticans (gas gangrene of the bowel)

C. botulinum:

- Anaerobic, gram-positive bacillus with subterminal spore
- Effect of toxin of Clostridium botulinum:

- o Blocks release of acetylcholine at neuromuscular junction
- o Botulinum toxin binds to acetylcholine receptors on the nerve terminals at neuromuscular junction, which results in blockage of release of the acetylcholine, leading to flaccid paralysis

C. tetani:

- Obligate anaerobic, gram-positive bacillus with terminal round spore (drum stick appearance)
- Tetanospasmin prevents the presynaptic release of inhibitory neurotransmitters glycine and GABA, which leads to spastic muscle contraction
- Clostridium tetani causes: Tetanus

Tetanus:

- Tetanus bacilli enter through injury (superficial abrasions, punctured wounds, road traffic accidents), surgery done without proper asepsis, neonates (following abortion/delivery)
- IP (Incubation period): 6-10 days
- Shorter the IP, graver is the prognosis
- Muscles of the face and jaw are often affected first (due to shorter distances for the toxin to reach the presynaptic terminals)
- First symptom – increase in the masseter tone leading to trismus or lock jaw
- Risus sardonicus (sustained spasm of the facial muscles)
- Opisthotonus (generalised spastic contraction of the extensor muscles)

E. COLI

Enterotoxigenic E.Coli:

- Most common cause for travelers' diarrhea: ETEC/Enterogenic E. coli
- Most common cause of travelers' diarrhea in 25-75% of cases
- Causes acute watery diarrhea in infants and adults

Enterohemorrhagic E. coli/EHEC:

- EHEC secretes a verocytotoxin/shiga-like toxin
- Shiga-like toxin causes capillary microangiopathy
- Causes hemorrhagic colitis and HUS

Enteropathogenic E. coli/EPEC:

- Causes infantile diarrhea (outbreaks)
- Important cause of infant diarrhea: EPEC/Enteropathogenic E. coli
- Nontoxigenic and noninvasive

YERSINIA PESTIS

Yersinia pestis:

- Gram-negative oval coccobacillus, often shows bipolar staining (ends of the bacilli stain darker than the central part) and pleomorphism (variable size and shapes) in older cultures
- Non-motile and capsulated
- Causes plague

Plague:

- Most common form of plague: Bubonic plague
- Transmitted by the bite of an infected rat flea
- IP: 2-7 days
- Buboes:
  - o Regional lymph nodes appear as tense, tender swellings
  - o Most common in inguinal region

BORDETELLA

Bordetella pertussis:

- Highly fastidious
- Very small
- Strict aerobe
- Gram-negative coccobacillus
- Grows best at 35-37 degree C
- Causes whooping cough

Whooping cough:

- IP of whooping cough: 7-10 days
- Clinical course of whooping cough/pertussis/100 days fever passes through 3 stages:
  - o Catarrhal stage
  - o Paroxysmal stage
  - o Convalescent stage

BRUCELLA

Brucella causes:

- Malta fever/Undulant fever/Mediterranean fever
- Fever has a typical remittent course, i.e., in between febrile periods (which lasts for weeks), there will be afebrile periods

TREPONEMA PALLIDUM

Treponema pallidum:

- Extremely thin bacilli and delicate with tapering ends
- Flexible, spirally coiled
- Cannot be visualized by light microscope

VDRL:

- A type of non-treponemal test/non-specific test/standard tests
- It is most widely used, simple and rapid serological test
- It is preferred for field studies and antenatal screening
- VDRL is positive in: Syphilis

OTHER BACTERIA

Proteus:

- Peritrichate flagella
- Urease positive (urease breaks down urea to form ammonia that damages renal epithelium and makes the urine alkaline)
- Effect of urease, produced by proteus:
  - o Urease hydrolyzes urea to ammonia, which results in alkalinization of urine
  - o Hence high prevalence of UTI in long-term catheterized individuals
- Alkaline urine predisposes to the deposition of phosphate, which leads to the formation of struvite calculi

Shigella:

- Most important agent of bacillary dysentery
- Nonmotile and not fermenting most sugars except mannitol
- Based on somatic O polysaccharide antigen, shigella is divided into 4 groups:
  - o Group A: S. dysenteriae
  - o Group B: S. flexneri
  - o Group C: S. boydii
  - o Group D: S. sonnei
- Most virulent type is:
  - o S. Dysentriae (group A): It does not ferment mannitol, in contrast to other species of Shigella, which are mannitol fermenters

Salmonella:

- Motile
- Non-sporing
- Non-capsulated
- Gram-negative bacilli
- Causes typhoid/Enteric fever
- Factor needed for growth: Tryptophan

Vibrio cholerae:

- Curved
- Gram-negative bacilli
- Actively motile by means of single polar flagellum
- Causes cholera
- Robert Koch isolated the organism in 1886, and names it as Komma bacillus (due to its characteristic curved or comma-shaped appearance)
- Special features of vibrio cholerae:
  - o Non-halophilic
  - o Can't grow in media with a concentration of NaCl more than 7%
  - o NaCl (0.5-1%) stimulates the growth, however, high concentrations of NaCl are inhibitory

Pseudomonas:

- Oxidase-positive
- Pigment producing
- Non-fermenting
- Gram-negative bacilli
- Major pathogen among the hospitalized patients and in patients with cystic fibrosis
- It causes:
  - o VAP (ventilator associated pneumonia)
  - o Malignant otitis externa
- Pseudomonas produces a number of pigments which diffuse freely into the surroundings
  - o Pyocyanin: Blue green pigment (produced only by P. aeruginosa)
  - o Pyorubin: Red color
  - o Pyomelanin: Brown black color

Hemophilus:

- Capsulated
- Pleomorphic
- Gram-negative bacilli that require special growth factors present in blood, such as factor X and V (Hemo means blood, philus means loving)
- H. ducreyi causes chancroid
- Factors required for growth:

- o Factor V and X
- o Hemophilus require these 2 accessory growth factors present in blood

***Mycobacterium tuberculosis*:**

- Non-motile, Non-sporing
- Non-capsulated
- Weakly gram-positive
- Straight or slightly curved rod-shaped bacteria
- Which are obligate aerobes (or microaerophilic)
- They sometimes show branching filamentous forms resembling fungal mycelium (myces means fungus)
- M. bacilli was discovered by: Robert Koch
  - o Robert Koch (1882) isolated the tubercle bacillus and proved its causative role in tuberculosis as it satisfies the Koch's postulates
- Factor responsible for acid fastness: Mycolic acid and cell wall
  - o Mycolic acid layer is the principal constituent, made up of long chain fatty acids attached to arabinogalactam
  - o It confers very low permeability to the cell wall and is responsible for acid fastness and also reduces the entry of most antibiotics
- Stain used for rapid diagnosis (screening) of M. bacilli: Auramine phenol stain
  - o Auramine phenol technique is a fluorescent technique, uses auramine phenol as primary stain, acid alcohol as decolorizer and potassium permanganate as counter stain
  - o The bacilli appear bright brilliant green against dark background
- Factor which promotes virulence: Cord factor

***Mycobacterium leprae*:**

- Strict aerobe
- Obligately intracellular bacilli
- Less acid fast as compared to tubercle bacilli
- Not cultivable either in artificial culture media or in tissue culture (so doesn't follow Koch's postulates)
- Generation time of M. leprae: 12-13 days
  - o Long generation time of 12-13 days as compared to 14 hours in tubercle bacillus and about 20 minutes for coliform bacilli
- M. leprae can be maintained in:
  - o Foot pad of mice (kept at low temperature, 20 degree C)
  - o Lepra bacilli can also be maintained in animals, such as nine banded armadillo (Dasypus novemcinctus)
- M. leprae spreads by:
  - o Prolonged contact with patients, who discharged bacilli in nasal secretions (nasal droplet infection)
    - – A sneeze from an untreated lepromatous leprosy patient may contain $>10^{10}$ lepra bacilli
  - o Contact transmission (skin):
    - – Direct contact from person to person
    - – Indirect contact with infected soil, fomites such as clothes and linens

***Borrelia*:**

- Poorly gram-stained (other spirochaetes do not take Gram stain)
- Lymes disease/erythema migrans is caused by: B. Burgdorferi
- Relapsing fever is caused by: B. Recurrentis
  - o Most reliable serological method for B. recurrentis is GlpQ (Glycerophosphodiester phosphodiesterase) assay

***Leptospira interrogans*:**

- Tightly and regularly coiled, with characteristic hooked ends (interrogans resembling interrogation/question marks)
- Spinning and translational movements
- Cannot be seen under light microscope (lepto means fine/thin)
- Leptospirosis is associated with:
  - o Rat
  - o Rice
  - o Rain
  - o The three most important epidemiological determinants for leptospirosis include exposure to rodents, rainfall and rice fields (3R's)

Mycoplasma:

- Also known as Eaton agent
- Prokaryotes, that are bounded by cell membrane
- As they lack cell wall, they show:
  - o Cellular pleomorphism
  - o Resistance to cell wall active antimicrobial agents (penicillins and cephalosporins)
- Appearance of colonies: Fried eggs colonies

Actinomycetes:

- Gram positive
- Growth usually results in formation of clumps (grains/sulfur granules)

Listeria:

- Genus received its current name, after the British pioneer of sterile surgery Joseph Lister, in 1940
- Gram-positive
- Rod-shaped
- Facultatively anaerobic
- Tumbling motility
- Test used: Anton's test
- Drug of choice for listerial meningitis: Ampicillin + Gentamicin

H. pylori:

- Gram-negative
- Spiral, flagellate bacillus
- Produces urease
  - o Urease protects it from acid by catalyzing conversion of urea to ammonia (buffer)
- Route of transmission of H. pylori: Man to man
  - o Faeco orally
  - o Orogastric route
- Most common cause of peptic ulcer

Rickettsia:

- Non-motile
- Gram-negative
- Nonspore forming
- Highly pleomorphic bacteria
- Rickettsial pox is caused by (vector: ticks): R. akari
- Q fever is caused by (only rickettsia NOT transmitted to humans by an arthropod): Coxialla burnetti

Chlamydia:

- Gram-negative
- Obligate intracellular bacteria (can grow inside a cell only)
- Cytoplasmic inclusion bodies by Giemsa stain
- C. Psittaci is acquired by inhalation of pigeon feces
- C. Trachomatis is acquired by sexual contact or vertically at birth
  - o Serotypes A-C causes trachoma
  - o Serotypes D-K causes genitourinary infections
  - o Serotype L1-L3 causes Lymphogranuloma venerum/ LGV

III. VIROLOGY

Viruses belonging to DNA group:

- Herpes viruses
- Hepadna viruses (Hepatitis B virus)
- Adenovirus
- Parvovirus
- Papillomavirus
- Polyomavirus (JC virus)
- Poxvirus (Smallpox, Molluscum contagiosum)

Viruses belonging to RNA group:

- Picornavirus (Poliovirus)
- Calicivirus (Hepatitis E virus)
- Reovirus (Rotavirus)
- Flavivirus (HCV, Yellow fever)
- Togavirus (Rubella)
- Retrovirus (HIV)
- Coronavirus
- Orthomyxovirus (Influenza virus)
- Paramyxovirus (Parainfluenza virus)
- Rhabdovirus (Rabies virus)
- Filovirus (Ebola virus)
- Arenavirus
- Bunyavirus
- Deltavirus (Hepatitis D virus)

Viruses belonging to herpes group:

- HSV-1 (Hereps labialis, Encephalitis)
- HSV-2 (Genital infections)
- Varicella zoster (Chickenpox, Shingles/Herpes zoster)

- EBV (Infectious mononucleosis, Burkitt's lymphoma, Naso-pharyngeal carcinoma, Oral hairy leukoplakia)
- CMV (Infection in AIDS)
- HHV-8 (Kaposi's sarcoma)

Polio:

- Polio virus (inside body) spreads by:
  - o Hematogenous route
  - o Neural route
- Most common manifestation of polio is: Subclinical infection (90%)
- Death in polio is mostly due to: Respiratory paralysis

Influenza virus:

- Antigenic drift (minor change): Small mutations in H and N
- Antigenic shift (major change)
- Bird flu virus is also known as: Avian flu influenza virus/ H5N1
- Swine flu (2009 outbreak) was due to: H1N1

Measles:

- Measles virus belongs to: Paramyxovirus
- Infectivity period of measles:
  - o 4 days before rash
  - o 5 days after rash appearance
- A rare, late neurological complication: SSPE (subacute sclerosing panencephalitis)

Mumps:

- Most common complication of mumps in post-pubertal males: Orchitis
- Special feature of mumps: One attacks gives life long immunity

Congenital rubella triad:

- Cataract
- Deafness
- Heart diseases (patent ductus arteriosus)

Rabies:

- Rabies virus is: Enveloped virus with ss RNA
- Negri bodies are pathognomic of: Rabies encephalitis
- They are present: Inside nerve cells
- For antemortem diagnosis: Immunofluorescence

Hepatitis:

- Special feature of hepatitis A virus (previously known as enterovirus 72): No chronic course
- Hepatitis B virus contains which enzyme: DNA dependent DNA polymerase (compare with HIV)
- Dane particle is: HBV
- HBV strain in India:
  - o Ayw
  - o Adr
- Maximum perinatal transmission risk for which hepatitis virus: HBV
- Serological marker of acute hepatitis B infection:
  - o HBsAg
  - o Core antibody (IgM anti-HBcAg)
- Epidemiological marker of Hepatitis B infection: HBsAg
- Indicator of high infectivity of hepatitis B infection:
  - o HBeAg
  - o HBV-DNA (indicator of intrahepatic viral replication)
- HCV belongs to which group: Flaviviridae
- Most common cause of post-transfusion hepatitis: HCV
- HEV is transmitted: Enterically/Faeco orally
- Highest mortality in pregnancy with hepatitis is with: HEV
- Hepatitis viruses spreading by faeco oral route are:
  - o HAV
  - o HEV

HIV:

- HIV consists of:
  - o 2 copies of ss RNA
  - o RNA dependent DNA polymerase (compare with HBV)
  - o Integrase
  - o Protease
- Seroconversion takes: 2-6 weeks
- Chances of transmission with accidental needle prick: 0.3%
- Retroviral sequence in host cell: RNA-DNA-RNA
- p24 antigen (used for early diagnosis) disappears after: 6-8 weeks of HIV infection
- CD4: CD8 ratio is: Reversed in HIV infection
- Window period: Time period between, infection to appearance of antibodies in serum
- During window period, ELISA and western blot are: Negative
- Most common cause of diarrhea in AIDS: Cryptosporodiosis (NOT cryptococcus)
- Most common cause of meningitis in AIDS: Cryptococcus
- Most common cause of oral ulcer in AIDS: Candida

- Most common cause of TB in AIDS in tropical countries: Mycobacterium TB
- Most common opportunistic infection in AIDS in India is: TB

Rotavirus:

- Double stranded RNA virus
- Non cultivable (does not grow in cell cultures)
- Detected by antigen in stools
- Most common cause of infantile diarrhea: Rotavirus

HPV:

- HPV with high oncogenic potential: HPV16, 18
- HPV causes warts, cervical intraepithelial neoplasia and cervical cancer

IV. MYCOLOGY

General facts:

- Fungi which are, spherical in tissue, but grow like molds, when cultures at room temperature are known as: Dimorphic fungi
- Fungal cell membrane is stained by:
    - o PAS
    - o Methanamine silver
- Fungi without sexual stage: Fungi imperfecti
- Culture media for fungi: Sabouraud's dextrose agar/SDA
- Non-culturable fungus: Rhinosporodium

Candida:

- Most common fungal infection in neutropenic patients: Candidiasis
- Reynolds Braude phenomenon is shown by: Candida
- Thrush is caused by: Candida (thrush is also known as oral candidiasis)

Dermatophytes infect:

- Skin
- Nail
- Hair

Cryptococcus:

- Cryptococcus has predilection for: Brain
- India ink (microscopy) wet mount is used for diagnosis of: Cryptococcus capsule
- Most common cause of acute meningitis in AIDS: Cryptococcus

Aspergillus:

- Hyphae in Aspergillus fumigates: Branching hyphae/Septate
- Portal of entry of Aspergillus fumigates: Lungs (can colonize the damaged bronchial tree, pulmonary cysts, cavities of patients with underlying lung tissue)

SECTION 2: PARASITOLOGY

I. NEMATODES/ROUNDWORM AND HOOKWORM

Ascaris lumbricoides/Giant roundworm:

- Eggs are visible in feces
- Bowel obstruction
- Iron deficiency

Wucheria bancrofti:

- Causes lymphatic filariasis by blocking lymphatic vessels
- Treated by DEC (DiEthylCarbamazine)

Loa Loa:

- Worm can be seen crawling in eye (conjunctiva)
- Causes Calabar swelling

Onchocerca volvulus:

- Causes river blindness
- Transmitted by female blackflies

Strongyloides stercoralis, Ancylostoma duodenale, Necator americanus (Hookworm):

- Larvae in soil penetrate the skin
- Iron deficiency anemia
- Cutaneous larva migrans

Toxocara canis:

- Visceral larva migrans
- Causes granulomas

Enterobius vermicularis/Pinworm:

- Food contaminated with eggs
- Causes anal pruritus

Dracunculus medinensis/Guinea worm:

- Largest nematode
- Causes inflammation and ulceration of skin

II. CESTODES/TAPEWORMS

Echinococcus granulosus/Dog tapeworm:

- Ingestion of eggs (in dog faeces) can result in cyst in liver (Hydatid cyst)

Taenia solium/Pork tapeworm:

- Causes cysticercosis and neurocysticercosis
- Ingestion of larvae encysted in undercooked pork
- Definitive host: Humans
- Intermediate host: Pig

III. TREMATODES

Schistosoma Japonicum:

- Host: Snails
- Causes: Urinary bladder carcinoma, hematuria

IV. MICROFILARIA

Microscopy of microfilaria:

- Microfilariae bancrofti: Tail tip free from nuclei
- Microfilariae malayi: Nuclei till tail tip

V. PROTOZOA

Entamoeba histolytica:

- Amoebic dysentery (bloody diarrhoea)
- Extra-intestinal: Amoebic liver abscess

Giardia lamblia/intestinalis:

- Foul smelling, non-bloody diarrhoea
- Treated by metronidazole

Trichomonas vaginalis:

- Trichominiasis presents with green colored, foul smelling discharge
- Motile trophozoites can be seen on wet mount

Leishmania donovani:

- Causes kala azar/visceral leishmaniasis
- Transmitted by sandfly

Cryptosporodium:

- Causes severe diarrhoea in AIDS

Naegleria fowleri:

- Causes rapidly fatal meningoencephalitis

Trypanosoma cruzi:

- Causes Chagas disease in South America
- Transmitted by Reduvid bug

Trypanosoma brucei:

- Causes African sleeping sickness
- Transmitted by TseTse fly

VI. PLASMODIA

4 types of plasmodia (Very Forward Medical Officer):

- Vivax
- Falciparum
- Malariae
- Ovale

P. vivax:

- Affects young RBCs (reticulocytes)
- Benign, tertian fever (fever every 3rd day; after 48 hours)
- Splenic rupture

P. falciparum:

- Affects all types of RBCs
- Multiple infestation of RBCs
- Malignant tertian malaria (fever every 3rd day; after 48 hours)
- Blackwater fever (Renal failure + DIC)
- Cerebral malaria

P. malariae:

- Affects mature RBCs
- Benign quartan fever (fever after 72 hours; every 4th day)

P. ovale:

- Rarest in India

8 CHAPTER

Biochemistry

I. ENZYMES

ISOENZYMES

Isoenzymes:

- Physically different forms of a same enzyme which catalyze same biochemical reaction
- Creatine kinase isoenzymes:
  - CK-1 (BB): Brain
  - CK-2 (MB): Heart
  - CK-3 (MM): Skeletal muscle
- Lactate dehydrogenase isoenzymes:
  - LDH-1 (HHHH): Heart
  - LDH-2 (HHHM): Blood (WBC)
  - LDH-3 (HHMM): Brain, kidney, lungs and pancreas
  - LDH-4 (HMMM): Muscle and liver
  - LDH-5 (MMMM): Muscle and liver

PARTS OF AN ENZYME

- Coenzyme is: Non protein organic compounds (all coenzyme are cofactors)
- Apoenzyme: Protein part
- Holoenzyme: Active enzyme

ENZYME INHIBITION

Competitive:

- Both inhibitor and substrate compete for the active site of enzyme
- Inhibitor binds with free enzyme, reversibly, to form enzyme-inhibitor complex, that is catalytically inactive
- Substrate cannot bind
- So a high concentration of substrate is required to offset the binding of inhibitor to the enzyme
- So K_m increases
- V_{max} remains same
- Inhibitor cannot bind with E-S complex

Non-competitive:

- Inhibitor and substrate have different sites of binding on enzyme
- Inhibitor doesn't bind at the active site
- Inhibitor can bind with Enzyme-substrate/E-S complex
- So K_m remains same
- V_{max} is lowered

II. AMINO ACID AND PROTEINS

AMINO ACIDS/AA

Important points:

- Total number of AA: 22
- 21st AA: Selenocysteine
- Essential AA: These are required in diet as they cannot be synthesized in the body
- Semi-essential AA: These are synthesized in the body but to some extent (Arginine and Histidine)
- Non-essential AA: These are not required in diet as they are synthesized in the body
- Most non polar amino acid is: Leucine
- Amino acid containing indole ring: Tryptophan
- Buffering action of blood is due to which amino acid: Histidine

ALIPHATIC AMINO ACIDS

Glycine:

- Formation of:
  - o Glutathione
  - o Creatine
  - o Haem

Alanine:

- Non-essential
- Alanine forms pyruvate (glucogenic)

Valine, Leucine and Isoleucine:

- Branched chain AA
- Defect in catabolism leads to MSUD

AROMATIC AMINO ACIDS

Phenyl-alanine/PA:

- Alanine + phenyl ring
- Essential AA

Tyrosine:

- Non-essential as it can be synthesized in body from PA
- Used for synthesis of:
  - o Melanin
  - o Thyroid hormones
  - o Catecholamines
    - – Dopamine
    - – Nor-epinephrine
    - – Epinephrine

Tryptophan:

- Forms:
  - o Serotonin (5-hydroxytryptamine)
  - o Melatonin
  - o Niacin (vitamin B3)

Histidine:

- Essential but semi-essential
- Maximum buffering capacity
- Catabolic end-product is glutamate

BASIC AMINO ACIDS/POSITIVELY CHARGED AA

Members:

- Arginine
- Lysine
- Histidine

Points:

- Arginine is most polar whereas Histidine is least polar

ACIDIC AMINO ACIDS

Members:

- Aspartate
- Glutamate

Points:

- Non-essential as they can be synthesized from TCA/Kreb's cycle intermediates

-OH CONTAINING AMINO ACIDS

Members:

- Serine
- Threonine
- Tyrosine

SULPHUR AMINO ACIDS/AA

Members:

- Cysteine
- Methionine

IMINO ACIDS

Proline:

- Unique structure helps proline in the fibrous structure of collagen

PROTEINS

Structure of proteins:

- Primary structure: Sequence of AA joined by peptide bond
- Secondary structure: folding of primary structure
  - o Alpha helix
  - o Beta sheet
- Tertiary structure: Single fully folded functional polypeptide chain
- Quaternary structure: Spatial relationship between individual polypeptide chains

AMINO ACID METABOLIC DEFECTS

Phenylketonuria/PKU:

- PKU is due to deficiency of: Phenylalanine hydroxylase/PAH
- PAH converts Phenyl Alanine/PA to Tyrosine
- Tyrosine becomes essential as it is not formed and there is excess of PA in body
- Excess PA is converted into Phenyl acetate and Phenyl pyruvate
- Mousy/musty odour of urine (due to Phenyl acetate)
- Treatment:
  - o Give Tyrosine as it is not formed
  - o Lifelong restriction of PA in diet

Alkaptonuria:

- It is due to deficiency of: Homogentisate oxidase
- Defect in catabolism of tyrosine and PA
- Urine turns black on exposure to air (due to oxidation of Homogentisic acid/HGA)
- Ochronosis: Deposition of black pigments (polymerization of HGA) in joints, collagenous tissue and cartilage
- Treatment:
  - o Vitamin C
  - o Restriction of tyrosine and PA

UREA CYCLE

Urea cycle/UC:

- Site of UC: Mitochondria and cytoplasm
- First 2 reactions of urea cycle occur in: Mitochondria (rest in cytoplasm)
- UC occurs in liver
- Carbamoyl Phosphate Synthetase-I is the rate limiting enzyme

III. CARBOHYDRATE

CLASSIFICATION

Monosaccharide:

- One carbohydrate unit
- Examples:
  - o Glucose
  - o Fructose
  - o Galactose

Disaccharide:

- 2 carbohydrate unit
- Examples:
  - o Sucrose
  - o Maltose
  - o Isomaltose
  - o Lactose

Oligosaccharide:

- Two to ten carbohydrates units
- Examples:
  - o Maltotriose

Polysaccharide:

- More than 10 carbohydrate units
- Homopolysaccharide
  - o Glycogen
  - o Starch
  - o Cellulose
  - o Chitin
  - o Inulin
- Heteropolysaccharide
  - o Hyaluronic acid
  - o Chondroitin sulfate
  - o Dermatan sulfate
  - o Keratin sulfate
  - o Heparan sulfate
  - o Heparin

GLYCOLYSIS/EMP PATHWAY/EMBDEN MEYERHOFF PATHWAY

Glycoslysis:

- Occurs in all the cell of the body
- Only pathway which can occur in both aerobic as well as anaerobic condition
- Occurs in cytoplasm
- Insulin activates it
- Catabolic process
- Tissue which depend on glucose as fuel:
  - o Brain
  - o Red blood cells
  - o Gastrointestinal tract
  - o Renal medulla
  - o Cancer cells
- Inhibitors of glycolysis:
  - o Iodoacetate
  - o Sodium fluoride
  - o Arsenate

KREB'S CYCLE/TCA CYCLE/CITRIC ACID CYCLE

Tricarboxylic acid cycle:

- First substrate of citric acid cycle is: Acetyl CoA which is derived from Pyruvate
- Amphibolic (both anabolic and catabolic) pathway
- Occurs in mitochondria
- Mature RBC lacks enzymes of: TCA/tricarboxylic acid cycle
- Occurs in aerobic condition
- Begins and ends with oxaloacetate
- First substance formed is Citric acid
- Inhibitors of TCA cycle:
  - o Malonate
  - o Fluoroacetate

GLUCONEOGENESIS

Gluconeogenesis:

- Occurs from:
  - o Glycerol
  - o Alanine
  - o Lactate
  - o Pyruvate
  - o Propionic acid
- Muscle cannot make use of glycogen as they lack: G-6-Phosphatase
- Catabolic pathway
- Occurs in:
  - o Liver and kidney
  - o In mitochondria and cytoplasm
- Activated by Glucagon
- Occurs in fasting state

HMP SHUNT

Hexose Mono Phosphate pathway:

- Minor pathway for production of glucose
- It is important as it produces: NADPH
- ATP produced in HMP shunt: No ATP is directly produced/ consumed
- Anabolic pathway
- Occurs in:
  - o Cytoplasm
  - o Liver, adipose tissue
- NADPH is used for:
  - o Fatty acid synthesis
  - o Steroid synthesis

- Important enzyme involved in NADPH synthesis: G6PD

GLYCOGEN STORAGE DISEASES

GSD:

- Most of the diseases in this category affect glycogenolysis (breakdown of glycogen is affected)
- Enzyme deficient in von-Gierke's disease (Type I GST): Glucose-6-phosphatase deficiency (affecting liver)
- Lactic acid and hyperuricemia is a feature of: Von-Gierke's disease (GST-I)
- Muscles are not involved in: Von-Gierke's disease (GST-I)
- Hypoglycemia, non-responsive to epinephrine is a feature of: Von-Gierke's disease (GST-I)

GALACTOSE METABOLISM

Galactosemia:

- Most common (of the 3) enzyme deficient in classical type galactosemia: GALT/Galactose-1-phosphate-uridyl transferase
- Cataract occurs because of the accumulation of: Galactilol/ Dulcitol
- Oil drop cataract
- Age of presentation is 1st week to 1st month of life
- Give lactose free diet (avoid breastfeeding)

ELECTRON TRANSPORT CHAIN

ETC:

- Electron transport chain is located in: Inner mitochondrial membrane
- Requires oxygen (aerobic)
- Components:
  - o 5 protein complexes (I - V)
  - o Coenzyme Q
  - o Cytochrome C
- Cyanide inhibits:
  - o Cytochrome oxidase (inhibits electron flow)
  - o Complex IV
  - o Cellular oxidation
- Cytochrome C oxidase/complex IV is inhibited by:
  - o Cyanide
  - o Carbon monoxide
  - o Hydrogen sulphide
- Complex III is inhibited by Phenformin (oral hypoglycemic agent)
- Uncoupler of oxidation and phosphorylation: 2, 4-Dinitrophenol/DNP

IV. FATS AND LIPIDS METABOLISM

FATTY ACIDS

Monosaturated fatty acids:

- One double bond present
- Oleic acid

Essential fatty acid/Polyunsaturated fatty acids/PUFAs:

- Essential in diet (as they are not synthesized in the body)
- Omega -3 category
  - o Cervonic acid
  - o Alpha-Linolenic acid
  - o Timnodonic acid
- Omega-6 category
  - o Linoleic acid
  - o Gamma-Linolenic acid
  - o Arachidonic acid
- Most essential fatty acid is: Linoleic acid (it can synthesize arachidonic acid)

CHOLESTEROL

Cholesterol synthesis:

- Rate limiting enzyme in cholesterol synthesis: HMG CoA reductase
- Anabolic pathway
- Occurs in Cytoplasm
- Insulin activates it
- Bile acids are derived from: Cholesterol

FATTY ACID/FA

Synthesis of FA:

- Synthesis of fatty acid occurs in: Cytosol
- Anabolic pathway
- Rate limiting step in fatty acid synthesis: Acetyl CoA carboxylase (contains biotin)
- Starting material: Acetyl CoA
- Activated by Insulin
- Main enzyme: FA synthase complex

Beta oxidation of fatty acids:

- Activation by Glucagon
- Occurs in:
  - o Mitochondria
  - o Liver, adipose tissues, muscles
- Occurs in starvation/fasting state
- Catabolic pathway
- Beta-oxidation of odd chain FA leads to production of propionyl CoA

Minor oxidation pathways:

- Alpha oxidation occurs in peroxisomes and endoplasmic reticulum
- Omega oxidation occurs in endoplasmic reticulum

KETONE BODIES/KB

KB:

- Ketone bodies are:
  - o Acetoacetate (primary KB)
  - o Acetone (secondary KB)
  - o Beta-hydroxyl butyrate (secondary KB; Most common)
- Rate limiting step in KB synthesis is HMG CoA synthase
- Ketone bodies are formed in liver
- KB are produced normally in minimal amounts but this amount is significantly raised during fasting and starvation
- Ketone bodies are product of:
  - o Increased lipolysis (Fatty acids metabolism)
  - o Increased acetyl CoA or decreased oxaloacetate
- Ketone bodies are normally produced from: Acetyl CoA
- Important feature of starvation ketosis: Ketone body formation without glycosuria

LIPOPROTEINS

Lipoproteins:

- HDL (high density)
- LDL (low density)
- VLDL (very low density)
- IDL (intermediate density)
- Chylomicron
- Most atherogenic lipoprotein: LDL (bad cholesterol)
- Lipoprotein with highest cholesterol content: LDL
- Lipoprotein with highest exogenous triglyceride content: Chylomicrons
- Lipoprotein which reverses cholesterol transport: HDL (good cholesterol)

V. NUCLEOTIDE

NUCLEOTIDE

Sugars:

- In RNA: Ribose
- In DNA: Deoxyribose

General information:

- Nucleoside: Nitrogenous base + Sugar
- Nucleotide: Nucleoside + phosphate
- Bases: Purine and Pyrimidine
- Purine:
  - o Adenine (A)
  - o Guanine (G)
- Pyrimidine:
  - o Cytosine (C)
  - o Uracil (U)
  - o Thymine (T)
- Bases in DNA: A, G, C and T (U is absent in DNA)
- Base present only in RNA and not in DNA: U

Purines:

- Occurs mainly in liver
- 2 pathways:
  - o De novo pathway
  - o Salvage pathway
- Key enzyme/Rate limiting enzyme for de novo synthesis pathway of purines: PRPP Glutamyl amido transferase
- Enzyme needed for salvage pathway of purines: HGPRTase
- End product of catabolism of purines in human beings: Uracil
- Reaction catalyzed by xanthine oxidase: XO converts hypoxanthine to xanthine and xanthine to uric acid

Pyrimidine:

- Rate limiting step for pyrimidine synthesis
  - o Prokaryotes: Aspartate transcarbamoylase
  - o Eukaryotes: Carbamoyl phosphate synthetase-II (CPS-II)

DNA

Bases in DNA:

- Adenine (A)
- Guanine (G)
- Cytosine (C)
- Thymine (T)

Differences between RNA and DNA:

- Deoxyribose sugar of DNA is replaced by a ribose moiety
- Instead of thymine (T), Uracil (U) is present in RNA
- Single strand in RNA and double strands in DNA

DNA REPLICATION

DNA replication:

- New synthesized strand is made in: 5' end →3' end direction
- Occurs in S-phase of cell cycle
- Okazaki fragments are formed during: Replication
- Function of helicase: DNA helix separation (zip opener)
- Semiconservative in nature (one of the parenteral strand is conserved during each cycle)
- Enzymes and functions (steps):
  - o Helicase: Separates strand
  - o Topo-isomerase: Relieve supercoils
  - o Single strand DNA binding proteins: Prevent rejoining of the 2 separated strands
  - o Primase: Synthesizes primers
  - o DNA polymerase III: Synthesize both leading and lagging strands
  - o DNA polymerase I: Remove RNA primers from both leading and lagging strands
  - o DNA ligase: Acts on lagging strand

TRANSLATION

Translation:

- Protein synthesis occurs mainly in: Ribosomes
- Fidelity enzyme in protein synthesis is: Amino acyl-tRNA synthetase
- Three steps:
  - o Initiation: Initiation codon is AUG
  - o Elongation
  - o Termination: When a stop codon is encountered on mRNA, then no AA will come

Codons:

- Codons are nucleotide triplets
- 4 nucleotide bases are employed to produce 3 base codons: A, U , C and G
- 6 characteristic of genetic code is:
  - o Triplet
  - o Universal
  - o Non-overlapping (A single codon have 1 amino acid)
  - o Degenerate (A single amino acid can have >1 representative codon)
  - o Non-punctuated
  - o Exhibit wobbling
- Stop codon is: Termination codon
  - o UAA
  - o UAG
  - o UGA
- Stop codons do not code for any amino acid

TECHNIQUES IN MOLECULAR BIOLOGY

Blotting types:

- Northern blot: RNA
- Southern blot: Detects DNA
- Western blot: Proteins (Antigen)

POLYMERASE CHAIN REACTION

PCR:

- Enzymatic DNA amplification
- In PCR, oligonucleotides build copies of the DNA using which enzyme: Heat stable polymerase (Taq1)
- Steps of PCR:
  - o Denaturation: 2 strands separated
  - o Annealing: Addition of primers (one for each strand)
  - o Extension/elongation: Polymerization or synthesis of DNA
- Substances required for PCR:
  - o 2 Primers
  - o Thermostable polymerase (taq polymerase)
  - o Magnesium
  - o ds-DNA
- Helpful in:
  - o Prenatal diagnosis: Beta-thalassemia, PKU
  - o Retroviral infections
  - o TB infections
  - o Detection of cancers
  - o Forensic medicine

VI. HEMOGLOBIN

Haem:

- Present in haemoglobin, myoglobin and cytochromes
- 'Haem' in haemoglobin is bonded to which amino acid: E7-Histidine
- Rate limiting step in haem synthesis is ALA synthase

Haem catabolism:

- Occurs in spleen, bone marrow (macrophages of reticulo-endothelial system)
- Steps:
  - o Bilirubin formation
  - o Hepatic uptake of bilirubin
  - o Bilirubin conjugation
  - o Disposal of bilirubin

Haemoglobin:

- Iron in haemoglobin is present in: Ferrous (Fe^{2+}) state
- Iron in haemoglobin is held by: Polar bonds
- Alpha2, Gamma2 is: Hb fetal

VII. VITAMINS

CLASS OF VITAMINS

Water soluble Vitamin:

- Vitamin B
- Vitamin C

Fat soluble Vitamin:

- Absorbed into intestinal lymphatics along with dietary lipids
- They cannot be excreted by kidneys
- Vitamin A, D, E and K

Functions:

- Vitamin which prevents lipid peroxidation: Vitamin E
- Vitamin needed for gamma carboxylation: Vitamin K
- Vitamin which is a post-translation modifier: Vitamin K

VITAMIN DEFICIENCIES

Features and deficient vitamins:

- Wernicke's Korsakoff syndrome is associated with deficiency of: Thiamine (B1)
- Consumption of egg (containing avidin) may lead to deficiency of: Biotin

- Methyl malonic aciduria is seen in deficiency of: Vitamin B_{12}/extrinsic factor of castle
- Scurvy is seen in deficiency of: Vitamin C

ENZYMES AND VITAMINS

Enzyme and related vitamins:

- Alpha-keto glutarate dehydrogenase is associated with: Thiamine (B1)
- RBC Transketolase is associated with: Thiamine (B1)
- **P**yruvate **c**arboxylase is associated with (PCB): **B**iotin
- **A**mino**t**ransferases is associated with (ATP): **P**yridoxine

9 CHAPTER

Toxicology

I. ANTIDOTE

Universal antidote (ATM):

- Animal charcoal:
  - o 2 parts
  - o Absorbs alkaloids
- Tannic acid:
  - o 1 part
  - o Precipitates alkaloids
- Magnesium oxide:
  - o 1 part
  - o Neutralizes acid without gas formation

II. METALLIC POISONS

Chronic mercury poisoning:

- Features:
  - o Erethism:
    - – Seen in persons working with mercury in mirror manufacturing firms
    - – Neuropsychiatric manifestations: Irritability, shyness, mental depression, loss of memory and insomnia
  - o Shaking palsy/Hatter's shake/glass blowers shake:
    - – Coarse, intentional tremors
  - o Mercurial lentis:
    - – Brown deposit of mercury through cornea on the anterior lens capsule
  - o Acrodynia/Pink disease:
    - – Acro means limbs; odynia means pain
    - – Hands and feet becomes puffy, pinkish, painful and paresthetic
  - o Hydrar gyrism:
    - – Fine tremors of the tongue, hands, arms etc.
- Acute mercury poisoning mainly involves: Kidney (PCT) causes proximal renal tubular necrosis
- Minimata disease: Contamination of fish with mercury (in Minimate Bay, Japan)

Arsenic poisoning:

- Findings on nails:
  - o Aldrich Mee's lines/leukoparonychia
  - o Transverse lines on nails
- 2 types of presentation:
  - o Fulminant type
  - o Gastroenteric type
- Gastroenteric type of Arsenic poisoning:

- o Most common type
- o Mimic Cholera poisoning
- o Stools are expelled frequently and involuntarily
- o Initially stools are dark coloured and stinking but later on becomes colorless, odourless and watery resembling rice water stools of cholera

- Skin changes associated with arsenic poisoning:
  - o Rain drop pigmentation: Finely mottled brown changes mostly on temples, eyelids and neck
  - o Rash resembling fading Measles rash
- Appearance of hair: Golden hair
- Arsenophagists:
  - o People who can tolerate high doses of arsenic as tonic or an aphrodisiac
  - o Tolerance of up to 0.3 gm or more in one dose
- Special feature of arsenic poisoning: Retardation of putrefaction and Delayed rigor
- Arsenic can be detected in: Completely decomposed bones, charred bodies, ash, hairs and nails
- Tests for arsenic poisoning:
  - o Marsh's test
  - o Reinsch's test
  - o Gutzeit test
- Treatment:
  - o Freshly prepared precipitated hydrated ferric chloride
  - o BAL is the antidote

Lead poisoning/plumbism/Saturnism:

- Inhalation of lead dust and fumes by makers of white lead, smelters, plumbers, glass polishers
- Features of lead poisoning/plumbism/saturnism (ABCDEF):
  - o Anemia (due to decreased RBC survival)
  - o Basophilia (punctate) of RBCs (dark blue spots in cytoplasm of RBCs)
  - o Burtonian/lead line in upper jaw
  - o Constipation and colic, Coproporphyrin in urine increased
  - o Death, wrist Drop and foot Drop
  - o Encephalopathy (in children)
  - o Facial pallor (most consistent sign)
- Burtonian line is seen at:
  - o Appears at the gingiva-tooth border
  - o Due to lead sulphide (after prolonged high level exposure)
- Early manifestation of chronic lead poisoning: Facial pallor
- Treatment: Combination of BAL + Calcium disodium versenare

III. CORROSIVE POISONS

Sulphuric acid:

- Strongest corrosive poison
- Brown to black streaks from angle of mouth present
- Effect of sulphuric acid poisoning on gastric mucosa:
  - o Stomach mucosa is stained black/scalded (Perforation of stomach is common)
  - o Blotting paper appearance of mucosa of stomach
- Fatal period for H_2SO_4: 18 to 24 hours
- Gastric lavage is contraindicated
- Vitriolage:
  - o Throwing of H_2SO_4 on other individual
  - o Comes under Sec. 320 IPC
  - o Affected part is washed with plenty of water and soap or sodium or potassium carbonate. Later a thick paste of magnesium oxide or carbonate is applied

Carbolic acid:

- Carbolic acid is also known as phenol
- Carboluria:
  - o Urine turns green or black on exposure to air/smoky green urine
  - o In the body phenol is partially oxidized to hydroquinone and pyrocatechol
  - o These are excreted in urine along with unchanged phenol
  - o The further oxidation of hydroquinone and pyrocatechol in the urine causes green coloration
- Appearance of stomach in carbolic acid poisoning: Mucous membrane is thickened and looks brownish and leathery (white leathery appearance)
- Special feature of carbolic acid poisoning: Retards putrefaction

IV. ORGANIC IRRITANT POISON

Abrus precatorius/Ratti:

- Seeds contain an active principle, a toxalbumin 'Abrin' (abrin resembles viper snake venom)
- Used as a cattle poison by making needles (sui)

Calotropis:

- Juice is introduced into uterus on an abortion sticks (criminal abortion)
- Also used as arrow poison
- Used to produce artificial bruises

For better preparation and success in AIIMS-NORCET Exam, download **'drkamalkvgroup'** mobile app from Google Playstore.

WhatsApp: +91 84 7000 4333

V. SNAKE

Snakes and nature of venom:

- Russells viper venom is: Hemolytic/Hemotoxic/vasculotoxic due to phosphotidase
- Cobra, Krait venom (elapidae family) is: Neurotoxic
- Sea/marine snake venom is: Myotoxic/Marked muscle weakness/polymyositis

For better preparation and success in AIIMS-NORCET Exam, download **'drkamalkvgroup'** mobile app from Google Playstore.

WhatsApp: +91 84 7000 4333

10 CHAPTER Fundamentals of Nursing

COMMON PROCEDURES

Checking axillary temperature:

- Read Hg level, while gently rotating thermometer at eye level
- Grasp thermometer/TM with thumb and forefinger and shake gently by snapping the wrist in a downward motion to move Hg to a level until reading lowers Hg level to 35.6 degrees C (DC)/96 degrees F (DF)
- Wait for 5 minutes and record the temperature
- Shake gently the TM so that the Hg level falls below 35 degrees C/95 degrees C
- Place the TM in disinfectant solution
- Note:
    - o Bath just before taking axillary temperature can alter the reading

Checking oral T:

- Ask the patient to open the mouth and gently place the TM under tongue in posterior sublingual pocket, lateral to the center of lower jaw
- Wait for 3 minutes and then read
- Note:
    - o Ask if patient has taken any hot/cold fluid. If yes, wait for 30 minutes to prevent false reading

Checking rectal T:

- Turn the patient to lateral position
- Lubricate the TM by putting Vaseline on its Hg tip
- Insert it about 4-5 cm into the anus and allow it to remain in for 3 minutes holding in place
- Remove and record temperature
- Axillary T: 97.6 DF
- Oral: 98.6 DF
- Rectal: 99.6 DF

Checking peripheral pulse:

- Place the second and/or third finger tips over radial A and press gently until the pulse is felt
- Determine pulse amplitude (reflects volume of blood ejected against arterial wall)
- Determine the rhythm
- When pulse has been detected, look at watch and count the pulse rate for 60 seconds
- Note:
    - o Ask if the patient has been mobilized/or has done any such motion within previous 15 minutes
    - o Anxiety or activity can alter pulse rate

Checking apical impulse:

- Expose sternum and left side of chest and position the diaphragm of the stethoscope over the point of maximal impulse (PMI) at the left 5th ICS, medial to mid-clavicular line
- If the heart beat is regular, count for 30 seconds and multiply by 2; if irregular, auscultate for full 1 minute

Checking respiration:

- Allow the patient to rest for at least 5 minutes
- Instruct the patient to stop talking during the procedure
- Promote the patient to keep hand over the abdomen or chest or place your hand over upper abdomen
- Watch complete respiratory cycle (I and E)
- Count the respirations for 1 minute
- Also record any abnormal breathing movement and regularity of chest movement

Measuring BP:

- Position the sphygmomanometer at the level of the heart with palm facing upwards
- Meniscus of Hg should be read at the eye level and more than 3 feet away
- Remove tight clothing and support the limb to be used for measurement
- Apply the correct-sized sphygmomanometer cuff 2.5 cm above the ante-cubital fossa in level with the heart
- Ensure the level of Hg in the SMM; it should be zero
- Close the valve of the pump; palpate the radial A gently with non-dominant hand and inflate the cuff, and note the point where the pulsations disappear (palpation method)
- Palpate the brachial A with fingers and place the SS in the ear and keep the diaphragm of SS over the brachial A gently; do not allow the SS to touch the clothing or the cuff
- Inflate the cuff until the Hg rises up to 2-3 mm Hg/s; the deflation should not be too fast or slow
- Note the point at which the sound become clear and louder; read the pressure to the closest even number and continue deflating the cuff and observe the point at which sounds disappear
- Do not show evidence of panic when a considerably low or high reading is obtained. Instead, doubly check
- To doubly check, repeat the procedure after a gap of 1 minute
- Note:
  - o Check for history of caffeine or smoking 30 minutes prior to BP measurement
  - o Recent meal, full bladder and cigarette smoking can affect BP
  - o Patient should rest for 5-15 minutes before recording BP in such cases
  - o Crossing of feet increases BP so feet should be kept flat
- C/I to BP measurement:
  - o Arm has I/V line
  - o Any injury to arm
  - o Arm has shunt or fistula for renal dialysis
  - o The side on which a breast/axillary surgery is done

Nasogastric tube insertion:

- Explain the procedure to the patient
- If possible, make the patient to sit in upright position for optimal neck/stomach alignment
- Examine nostrils for deformity/obstruction
- Measure tubing from bridge of nose to earlobe, then to the point halfway between the end of the sternum and the navel
- This is done to insert the appropriate size to prevent coiling of the tube inside the GIT
- Lubricate 2-4 inches of tube with lubricant (preferably 2% xylocaine)
- Pass tube via either snare posteriorly, past the pharynx into the esophagus and then into the stomach
- Instruct the patient to swallow (may offer water) an advance the tube as the patient swallows; swallowing of small sips of water may enhance passage of tube into esophagus
- If resistance is met, rotate tube slowly downward advancement; do not force
- Withdraw the tube immediately, if changes occur in patient's respiratory status, if tube coils in mouth; if the patient begins to cough
- Advance tube until the mark is reached
- Check for placement by attaching syringe to the free end of the tube, aspirate sample of gastric contents; obtain X-ray to verify placement before instilling any feedings/medication or if you have concern about the placement of the tube
- Secure tube with tape
- Monitor vital signs of the patient

Nasogastric tube feeding:

- Assist the patient to a Fowler's position in bed or sitting position on chair
- If sitting position is contraindicated, a slightly elevated right side lying position is acceptable
- Assess the tube placement by attaching the syringe to open end of the tube and aspirate gastric secretion
- Before administering the feeding, check the temperature and texture of the feed
- Pinch the loop and remove the syringe from the tube and rinse it
- Connect the barrel of the syringe to the pinched or clamped nasogastric tube

- Allow the feeding to flow slowly at the prescribed rate and pinch or clamp the tube, stop the feed if patient feels discomfort
- At the end of the feed, flush the tube with a measured amount of water
- Pinch the loop of the tube and remove the syringe and close the tube with plunger
- Allow the patient in semi-Fowler's position for 5-10 minutes

Surgical dressing:

- Before starting procedure, make sure the sweeping and the mopping of the ward is completed
- Provide privacy to the patient
- Wear unsterile gloves and remove the old dressing. Keep the adherent gauze well in place
- Remove the gloves and wear sterile gloves before dressing proper
- Soak the adherent gauze with saline and remove it with artery clamp/forcep
- Once the surgical site is exposed dress it
- Clean the wound (with spirit)
- Use separate cotton ball for each stroke
- Use dry gauze to clean the incision
- Apply betadine ointment
- Apply the sterile dressing to incision/drain site
- Secure dressing with bandage or adhesive

SPECIMEN COLLECTION

Collection of blood specimen:

- Positioning:
  - o Make the patient to be seated comfortably or supine position
  - o Assist the patient with the arm extended to form a straight line from shoulder to wrist
- Select the appropriate vein for venipuncture
- Applying the tourniquet:
  - o Apply tourniquet 3-4 inches (8-10 cm) above the collection site; never leave the tourniquet on for over 1 minute
  - o If a tourniquet is used for preliminary vein selection, release it and reapply after 2 minutes
- Selection of the vein:
  - o Feel the vein using the tip of the finger and detect the direction, depth and size of the vein
  - o Massage the limb from wrist to elbow; tell the patient to make a fist; if the vein is not prominent, try the other arm
- Disinfect the selected site:
  - o Clean the puncture site by making a smooth circular pass over the site with spirit swab, moving in an outward spiral from the zone of penetration
  - o Allow the skin to dry before penetration
- Hold the syringe with the bevel of needle facing upwards
- Advance the needle into the patient vein, with the patient's arm in a downward position
- As blood come into view in syringe, withdraw the plunger of the syringe softly and steady suction until the required sample is obtained
- Release the tourniquet and ask the patient to open the fist
- Place a dry gauze over the puncture site and remove the needle
- Immediately apply slight pressure; ask the patient to apply pressure for at least 2 minutes
- Transfer blood into appropriate blood specimen bottles or tubes as soon as possible using needleless syringe
- The container or tube containing an additive should be gently inverted 5-8 times or shaking the specimen container by making figure of 8
- Dispose the syringe and needle into appropriate containers
- Label all tubes or specimen bottles with patient details

Collection of blood for culture:

- Definition:
  - o A blood culture is a collection and inoculation of blood into culture medium with the aim of growing pathogenic bacteria for diagnostic purpose
- Purpose:
  - o To identify the type of bacteria present and specific type of antibiotics to use to eradicate the bacteria
- Same steps as in venipuncture and collection of blood sample
- After blood is taken, remove the needle from the syringe, discard into sharps container

- From the syringe, distribute blood equally into aerobic and anaerobic labeled sample container
- Gently rotate the bottles to mix the blood and the broth (do not shake vigorously) and send the specimen to respective laboratories

Arterial blood collection:

- ABG (arterial blood gases) are diagnostic tests performed on blood taken from an artery
- ABG are done to evaluate oxygenation and acid-base balance in the body
- Check the patient coagulation factors and platelet count before starting the procedure
- Feel for the radial pulses on both the wrists to determine which will be better side, for withdrawing blood
- Perform Allen's test on the hand, which has been selected for the procedure
- Allen test:
  - o Hand is elevated and fist is made for about 30 seconds
  - o Pressure is applied over the ulnar A and radial A so as to occlude both of them
  - o Still elevated, the hand is then opened
  - o Hand should appear blanched (pallor can be observed at the finger nails
  - o Ulnar pressure is released and the color should return in 7 seconds
  - o Inference:
    - – Ulnar A supply to the hand is sufficient and it is safe to cannulate/prick the radial A
    - – If the color does not return after 7-10 seconds, then the test is considered negative and the ulnar A supply to the hand is not sufficient
    - – The radial A therefore cannot be safely pricked/ cannulated
- Put sterile gloves and anesthetize the puncture site with 2% xylocaine
- The heparinized syringe should be used to withdraw the blood sample
- Puncture the skin about 5-10 mm distal to the finger directly over the artery, the puncture angle should be approximately 45 degrees towards the direction of the blood flow
- Slowly advance the needle and syringe with one hand, while continuing to palpate the artery with other hand; when a flash of arterial blood is observed in the hub of the needle, do not advance the needle further
- While holding the syringe and the needle motionless with one hand, gently pull back on the plunger of the syringe with the other hand to allow the syringe to fill
- If the needed amount of blood has been obtained, one should remove the needle and syringe rapidly, and press down the puncture site with sterile gauze for about 5 minutes
- If any bleeding occurs at the end of this time, pressure should be maintained until no further bleeding occurs. Press longer, if the patient has any bleeding tendencies
- If any air bubbles are present in the syringe, it is to be removed immediately and recap the needle
- Send the sample to blood gas analyzer
- Note:
  - o Arterial blood will pulsate whereas blood from vein does not
  - o Arterial blood is brighter red (if oxygenation is adequate) than blood from a vein

Measurement of capillary blood glucose:

- Helps to observe immediate and daily levels of blood glucose control and dose adjustments
- Clean the fingertip with the alcohol swab where must prick
- Allow the area to dry and prick the fingertip with the use of single use lancet
- Take a blood sample from the pricking site of the finger, ensuring the site of the piercing is rotated
- Finger bleed without assistance or may need assistance by exploiting to form a droplet of blood, which is large enough to cover the test pad
- Apply the blood to the testing strip; some test strips are hydrophilic and are dosed/filled from the side and not dropped directly onto the strip
- Dispose the lancet into the puncture proof sharps container
- Record value immediately after the test has been done

Collection of urine specimen:

- Label specimen containers or bottles before the client voids (reduce handling after the container or bottle is contaminated)
- Note on the specimen label, if the female client is menstruating at that time (one of the tests routinely performed is a test for blood in the urine. If the female patient is menstruating at the time of collection, a false +ve test will be obtained)
- To avoid contamination and necessity of collecting another specimen, soap and water cleansing of the genitals immediately preceding the collection of samples is supported (bacteria are normally +nt in genitals)
- Maintain body substances precautions, when collecting all types of urine specimen

- Take the sample in the morning (represents the urine that was collected in the bladder at night)

Collection of single-voided specimen:

- Prefer MSU

Collection of throat swab:

- Make the patient sit in the bed or raise the head end of the bed, if not C/I
- Ask the patient to tilt head backward and open mouth, stretch the tongue out
- Visualize the tongue and throat by using torch light
- Use tongue spatula to press the tongue downward to the floor of the mouth
- Use sterile cotton swab to wipe down both of the tonsillar arches and the posterior nasopharynx, without touching the side of the mouth
- Place the swab in labeled culture tube and close the tube

Wound swab collection:

- Wear gloves and open the dressing
- Remove the solid dressing materials with an artery forceps
- Wear another pair of gloves
- Remove the swab stick from the collection kit or the tube and do not touch the soft tip or lay down the swab
- Take the swab before cleaning the wound
- Use a zig-zag motion whilst simultaneously rotating between fingers
- Place the swab into the labeled test tube and the tip of the swab is visible below the tube label; recap the container

OXYGEN THERAPY

Administration of oxygen therapy:

- Oxygen is supplemented at higher percentages than what is available in atmospheric air
- Purpose:
  - o To relieve dyspnea
  - o To reduce or prevent hypoxemia and hypoxia
  - o To alleviate the struggle associated with breathing
- Sources of oxygen: Therapeutic O_2 is available from two sources:
  - o Wall outlets (central supply)
  - o Oxygen cylinders
- Alerts:
  - o Explain the patient the dangers of lighting matches or smoking cigarettes, cigars etc.
  - o Do not use oil on oxygen equipment as oil can ignite if exposed to O_2
- O_2 is turned on before the mask is applied to the patient
- Maintain a constant O_2 concentration for the patient to breathe; monitor equipment at regular intervals
- Watch for respiratory depression or distress
- Provide frequent mouth care
- Make sure the O_2 contains proper humidification
- One should not abruptly discontinue O_2 given in medium-to-high concentrations (above 30%)
- Gradually decrease in stages and monitor the patient's ABG or O_2 saturation level
- Always be careful when you give high levels of O_2 to patients with COPD
- Elevated levels of O_2 in the patient's body can depress the stimulus to breathe

O_2 administration:

- 2 methods:
  - o Nasal cannula
  - o Face mask

Nasal cannula/prongs method:

- Attach the flowmeter into the wall outlet or oxygen cylinder
- Fill humidifier about one-third with sterile water or boiled water
- Attach the cannula with the connecting tubing to the adapter, on the humidifier
- Test flow by setting flowmeter at 2-3 L/min and check the flow on hand
- Adjust the flowmeter's setting as per order
- Insert the nasal cannula into patient's nostrils, adjusting the tubing behind the patient's ear and slide the plastic adapter under the patient's chin
- Encourage the patient to breathe through the nose rather than the mouth and expire from the mouth
- Assess the patient's response to oxygen and comfort level

OXYGEN DELIVERY SYSTEM

High-flow system:

- Delivers a constant % of oxygen
- Independent of patient's breathing
- Venturi mask, T-piece etc.

Low-flow system:

- Does not provide a constant fraction of inspired oxygen
- Such system contributes only partially to the gas which is inhaled by the patient
- Simple mask, nasal cannula etc.

INJECTION PREPARATION

Single dose ampoule:

- Inspect the solution for cloudiness or particulate matter; if this is present, discard it
- Tap the neck of the ampoule gently
- Cover the neck of the ampoule with a sterile topical swab and snap it open
- Inspect the solution for glass fragments; if present, discard
- Withdraw the required amount of solution, tilting the ampoule if necessary
- Replace the sheath on the needle and tap the syringe to dislodge any air bubbles; expel air

Single-dose ampoule powder preparation:

- Open the ampoule as discussed before
- Inject the correct diluents slowly into the powder within the ampoule
- Agitate the ampoule
- Inspect the contents, withdraw into syringe as discussed before

Multidose vial powder preparation:

- Remove the tamper evident seal and clean the rubber septum with an antiseptic
- Let it air dry for at least 30 seconds
- 2 methods:
  - o Restitution method
  - o Reconstitution method

Restitution method:

- Insert a 21G needle into the cap to vent the bottle
- Inject the correct diluent slowly into the powder within the vial
- Remove the needle and the syringe
- Place a sterile topical swab over the venting needle and shake to dissolve the powder
- Inspect the solution for cloudiness or particulate matter. If found then discard

Reconstitution method:

- Draw into the syringe, a volume of air equivalent to the required volume of diluent to be drawn up
- Insert the needle into the diluent solution
- Invert the vial of diluent; keep the needle into the solution; slowly depress the plunger to push the air into the vial
- Release the plunger, so that the diluent solution flows back into the syringe. If a large volume of solution is to be withdrawn, then use a push pull technique
- Inject the diluents into the vial containing powder, keeping the tip of the needle above the level of the solution in the vial
- Release the plunger; the syringe will fill with the air, which has been displaced by the solution
- With the needle and syringe in place, gently swirl the vial to dissolve the powder
- Inspect the solution for cloudiness or particulate matter
- Discard the vial, if this is noted

Withdrawal of medication from vial:

- Withdraw the prescribed amount of drug
- Inspect for pieces of rubber, which may have cored out of the cap
- Remove air from the syringe without spraying in air
- Either inject back the air into the vial or replace the sheath on the needle and tap the syringe to dislodge any air bubble; expel air

ADMINISTRATION OF INJECTIONS

Route and angle of injection:

- Intradermal: 10-15 degrees
- I/V: 25 degrees
- S/C: 45 degrees
- I/M: 90 degrees

Administration of subcutaneous injection:

- A S/C injection is a method of drug administration into the S/C tissue
- Up to 2 ml of a drug solution can be injected directly beneath the skin
- With the S/C route, a small thin needle is inserted beneath the skin and the drug is injected slowly
- The drug moves from the small blood vessels into the bloodstream
- Sites:
  - o Outer aspect of upper arm
  - o Posterior chest wall below scapula
  - o Anterior abdominal wall from below the breast to iliac crest
  - o Anterior and lateral aspect of the thigh
- Assess the injection site for any signs of inflammation, edema, infection and skin lesions
- Choose the correct needle size
- Clean the injection site with a swab saturated with 70% isopropyl alcohol
- Gently pinch the skin up into a fold
- Insert the needle into the skin at an angle of 45% and release the grasped skin; inject the drug slowly
- Withdraw the needle rapidly; apply pressure to any bleeding point; do not rub

Administration of intradermal injections:

- Administration of injection with an angle of 5-15 degree into the dermal layer of the skin
- Purpose: Certain medication may be injected intradermally to test the allergy
- Assess the injection site for any signs of inflammation, edema, infection and skin lesions
- Clean the injection site with a swab saturated with 70% isopropyl alcohol
- Stretch the skin around the injection site
- Holding the needle level up at an angle of 5-15 degree, slowly plunge into the skin and administer the drug
- Notice that, while injecting the medication, small bleb approximately 6 mm in diameter appears on the skin surface
- Withdraw the needle, while applying alcohol swab or gauze gently over site rapidly
- Apply gentle pressure, do not massage site
- Use blue ink pen and draw a circle round perimeter of injection site
- Observe the patient for 3-5 minutes for any allergic reactions

Intramuscular injection:

- Provides faster medication absorption than the subcutaneous route b/c of a greater muscular vascularity
- Sites:
  - o Deltoid
  - o Vastus lateralis
  - o Ventrogluteal
  - o Dorsogluteal

Upper arm:

- 5 cm distal to the acromion and 4 cm proximal of insertion of deltoid
- Prevent damage to the circumflex humeral nerve

Gluteal region:

- Upper outer quadrant is preferred
- Prevent damage to superior and inferior gluteal vessels and sciatic N

Dorsogluteal

- Right gluteal area:
  - o Keep ball of the left index finger just above the greater trochanter and the tip of the index finger pointing over the ASIS, the middle finger at right angle to the index finger and pointing towards iliac crest

Lateral aspect of thigh:

- Ideal site as no vessels or N come in the way
- Cleanse hand with alcoholic hand rub
- Assess the site for inflammation, edema, infection and skin lesions
- Clean the injection site with a swab saturated with 70% isopropyl alcohol for 30 seconds and allow it to dry for 30 seconds
- Stretch the skin around injection site

- Holding the needle at an angle of 90 degree, quickly plunge into the skin
- Pull back the plunger; if no blood is aspirated, depress the plunger at approximately 1 ml every 10 seconds and inject the drug slowly
- If blood appears, withdraw the needle completely, replace it and begin again; explain to the patient what has occurred
- Wait for 10 seconds before withdrawing needle
- Withdraw the needle rapidly; apply pressure to any bleeding point

Z-track method:

- Preferred site is I/M
- Zigzag path seals the needle track when the tissue planes slide across each other thus the medicine cannot escape from the muscle tissue
- This also minimizes the local skin irritation as the medication is sealed in the muscle plane

INTRAVENOUS INJECTIONS

Administration of intravenous injections:

- Parenteral administration of bolus medication directly into the vein

3 methods of I/V injection administration:

- Continuous infusion
- Intermittent infusion
- Direct intermittent injection

Continuous infusion:

- I/V delivery of medication/fluid at a constant rate over a prescribed time period (24 hours to days), to achieve a controlled therapeutic response

Intermittent infusion:

- Administration of a small volume infusion, i.e., 50-250 mL over a period of 20 minutes to 2 hours

Direct intermittent injection:

- Injection of a drug from a syringe into the injection port of the administration set or directly into a vascular access device

Intravenous cannulation:

- Position the patient with the arm extended to form a straight line from shoulder to wrist joint
- Wash hands with bactericidal soap and water or bactericidal alcohol hand rub
- Select the appropriate vein for I/V cannulation; it should be straighter and more prominent; e.g., the vein in the forearm or dorsum of the hand
- Palpate the vessel; apply a tourniquet 7-10 cm above the site gently and it should not be too tight
- Put on gloves and clean the skin over selected site with alcohol swab
- Hold patient's hand with your non-dominant, using your thumb to keep skin taut and anchor vein
- Remove the protective sleeve from the needle taking care not to touch it
- Hold the cannula in your dominant hand, stretch the skin over the vein to anchor the vein with your non-dominant hand (do not re-palpate the vein)
- The needle is inserted bevel up; the initial angle of entry should be approximately 15-30 degrees
- Observe the blood in flashback chamber
- Lower the cannula slightly to ensure that the cannula enters the lumen in the vessel and does not pierce it
- Gently advance the cannula over the needle whilst withdrawing the guide, noting secondary flashback along the cannula
- Release the tourniquet and apply pressure over the vein (beyond the cannula tip); remove white cap from the needle
- Remove the needle from the cannula; attach the white lock cap and dispose of into a sharp container
- Secure the cannula with an appropriate dressing and flush the cannula with 2-5 ml of 0.9% NaCl or attach an I/V giving set and fluid
- Do not attempt venipuncture more than twice

I/V infusion:

- Prepare I/V solution and tubing:
  - o Maintain aseptic technique when opening sterile packages and I/V solution
  - o Clamp tubing by using roller clamp, uncap spike and insert into entry site on bag
  - o Squeeze dip chamber and allow it to fill at least one-third to halfway
  - o Remove cap at the end of the tubing, release clamp, allow fluid to move through tubing, allow fluid to flow until all air bubbles have disappeared

- o Close clamp and recap end of tubing, maintaining sterility of setup
- o Apply label if medication has been added to container
- o Hang on I/V stand
- Selection the site for venipuncture:
  - o Select an appropriate site and palpate accessible vein
  - o Apply a tourniquet 5-6 inches above the venipuncture site to obstruct the venous blood flow and distend the vein
- Palpate the vein:
  - o Ask the patient to open and close the fist
  - o Observe and palpate for a suitable vein
- If the vein cannot be felt and seen, release the tourniquet and have the patient lower arm below the level of the heart to fill the veins; reapply tourniquet and gently tap over the vein
- Else after removing tourniquet, place warm and moist compress over the intended vein for 10-15 minutes

Preparing for venipuncture:

- Put on the gloves
- Cleanse the skin over the entry site with spirit swab using a circular lotion to move away from the center to outward
- Place a non-dominant hand about 1-2 inches below entry site to hold the skin taut against the vein
- Avoid touching the prepared area

Puncturing the vein and withdrawing blood:

- Enter the skin gently with the catheter/cannula held by the hub in the dominant hand, bevel side up, at an angle of 15-30 degrees
- Catheter may be inserted from directly over the vein or the side of the vein
- While following the course of the vein, advance the needle or catheter into the vein
- A sensation can be felt when needle enters the vein
- When the blood returns through the lumen of the needle or the flashback chamber of the catheter, advance the device 1/8 to ¼ inch further into the vein
- Connecting to the tube and stabilizing the catheter on the skin:
  - o Release the tourniquet
  - o Quickly remove protective cap from the I/V tubing
- Attach the tubing to the catheter
- Stabilize the catheter with non-dominant hand
- Starting flow:
  - o Release the clamp on the tubing
  - o Start flow of solution promptly
- Examine the drip of solution and the tissue around the entry site for any signs of infiltration
- Fasten the catheter/needle and apply dressing:
  - o Secure the catheter/needle with tape
  - o Loop the tubing near the site of entry

I/V FLUIDS

Types:

- Hypotonic:
  - o Lower concentration of than body fluids
  - o NaCl 0.3%
- Isotonic: Same concentration as body fluids
  - o NaCl 0.9%
  - o Plain RL
  - o D5W
- Hypertonic: Higher concentration than the body fluids
  - o D10W
  - o D50W

For better preparation and success in AIIMS-NORCET Exam, download **'drkamalkvgroup'** mobile app from Google Playstore.

WhatsApp: +91 84 7000 4333

LOCAL ANESTHETIC INJECTION

Local anesthetic/LA injection:

- Explain the procedure to the patient
- Fill the syringe with LA
- Do xylocaine sensitivity (intradermal)

- LA can be used with or without adrenaline
- This combination is C/I in fingers, toes, ears and penis since it causes vasospasm of the end arteries to result in gangrene of these parts
- Action of adrenaline is to constrict the blood vessels so that bleeding is diminished and the duration of LA is prolonged
- Inject the LA subcutaneously, which will block small S/C nerves and their N endings
- Aspirate before injecting, to confirm that the needle is not in a vessel
- Always keep the needle moving (withdraw)
- Wait for few minutes for the effect of LA to come
- Till then wash your hands and wear gloves

INSULIN INJECTION

Administration of insulin injections:

- Insulin should be given as injection b/c it is a protein and therefore would be broken down and destroyed in GIT

Route of administration:

- Subcutaneous/hypodermic (into the subcutaneous tissue)
- Needle:
  - o 25-27 G
  - o 5/8 to ½ inch
- Position: 45 – 90 degrees
- Syringes:
  - o 1 ml for 100 U of insulin
  - o 1 ml for 40 U of insulin
- Advantages of giving in S/C tissue:
  - o Minimal risk of hitting blood vessel
  - o Allows slower absorption
  - o Allows slower, more sustained drug administration than I/M injection
- Cautions:
  - o Do not give injection in scarred areas, in moles, inflamed tissue
  - o Do not massage after administration
- Sites:
  - o Outer aspect of upper arm
  - o Anterior thigh
  - o Loose tissue of the lower abdomen
  - o Upper hips
  - o Buttock
  - o Upper back
- Procedure:
  - o Obtain an insulin syringe
  - o Pick up the vial and verify the type of insulin, which is prescribed
- Check the patient's most recent blood glucose, if in case of doubt, always recheck and reassess
- Wipe the insulin vial with a sterile gauze alcohol pad, if the insulin is cloudy, roll between palms of your hands
- Withdraw the appropriate type and amount of insulin
- Pull back the barrel of the syringe to draw in a volume of the ordered medication dose; holding the vial between the thumb and fingers of non-dominant hand, insert the needle through the rubber stopper into the air space, not the solution
- Invert the vial and withdraw the ordered dose of medication by pulling back on the plunger; make sure the needle is in the solution to be withdrawn
- Expel air bubbles and adjust the dose
- Remove needle from vial and cover the needle with guard using one hand or scoop method
- Administer by S/C route; remember never massage the insulin injection site

Insulin pen:

- Wash hands
- Choose and clean injection site
- Screw pen needle firmly onto pen
- Prime: Dial '2' units
- Hold upright; remove air by pressing the plunger; repeat 'prime' if no insulin shows at the end of the needle
- Dial number of units to be administered as per order
- Pinch up the skin
- Push the needle at an angle of 90 degrees
- Release pinched skin
- Leave the needle in the skin and keep pressing the button for 5-10 seconds
- Remove and dispose pen needle

URINARY CATHETERIZATION

Male urinary catheterization:

- Provide privacy to the patient and explain the procedure to the patient
- If applicable, ensure the patient has washed genital area using soap and water, and if necessary, assist using non-sterile gloves
- Place the Mackintosh under patient's buttock
- Wash hand using bactericidal soap and water or bactericidal alcohol hand rub
- Wear sterile gloves
- If patient is uncircumcised, it would be necessary to retract the prepuce with non-dominant hand
- Hold penis with a gauze swab; clean penis with sterile NS 0.9% or antiseptic solution with dominant hand
- Instill 11 ml of anesthetic gel into urethral meatus, still holding penis with non-dominant hand, gently compress penis behind glans to retain gel and massage gel along urethra
- Allow for 5 minutes for anesthetic gel to take effect
- Pick up catheter by holding inner wrapper and expose tip of catheter 1-2 inches (5 cm)
- The remaining length should lie in the container, which should be placed between patient's leg
- Holding penis at an angle of 60-90 degrees to body, gently insert into meatus and pass along the urethra maintaining gentle pressure
- Advance the catheter 6-8 cm and inflate the balloon by pushing NS through a syringe, having ensured that the catheter is draining adequately in urobag
- Secure to lower abdomen
- If resistance is met while passing catheter, tell the patient to cough
- It may reduce pressure on the external sphincter and ease the passage of the catheter
- Force should never be used

Female urinary catheterization:

- Provide privacy to the patient and explain the procedure to the patient
- If applicable, ensure the patient has washed genital area using soap and water, and if necessary, assist using non-sterile gloves
- Place the Mackintosh under patient's buttock
- Wash hand using bactericidal soap and water or bactericidal alcohol hand rub
- Wear sterile gloves
- Place sterile towels in patient's thighs and under buttocks in transversely and expose genital area
- With thumb and one finger of your non-dominant hand, spread labia and identify meatus; be prepared to maintain separation of labia with non-dominant hand until urine is flowing well and continuously
- Using cotton balls held with forceps in dominant hand, clean area around the urethral meatus with sterile NS 0.9% or antiseptic solution
- Instill 3-6 ml of anesthetic gel into urethral meatus
- Allow for 5 minutes for anesthetic gel to take effect
- Pick up catheter in dominant hand, by holding inner wrapper and expose tip of catheter 1-2 inches (5 cm)
- The remaining length should lie in the container, which should be placed between patient's leg
- Gently insert into meatus and pass along the urethra maintaining gentle pressure, until urine flows
- Inflate the balloon by pushing NS through a syringe, having ensured that the catheter is draining adequately in urobag
- Tie the urobag to the bed and secure the catheter to the thigh (in males, it is secured to the lower abdomen so that the catheter does not pull the penis downward)
- Force should never be used

IRRIGATION

Urinary bladder irrigation:

- A procedure in which instillation of a solution is done into the bladder to provide cleansing
- Purpose:
    - o To maintain the patency of retention catheter by removing bladder sediment or blood clots

- o To clean the bladder
- 2 methods:
  - o Closed method
  - o Continuous method

Closed method:

- If the patient is on urinary catheter, detach the urobag from the catheter and cover the tip with sterile gauze pieces
- Load the bladder wash syringe with solution (NS or sterile water) and expel the air, attach the tip of the syringe into the catheter
- Install the solution slowly into the bladder usually not more than 80-100 cc at a time
- Remove the syringe and allow the urine to drain into the kidney tray
- Repeat installing and emptying till the return flow is clean
- Connect the catheter to the urobag again

Continuous method:

- Prepare the bladder irrigation solution as prepared for I/V infusion, hang the solution bottle on irrigation stand at a height of about 5-6 inches above the level of meatus and allow expelling air from the irrigation set
- Clean the catheter and urobag junction with alcohol swab
- Wear gloves
- Connect the tubing to 3-way urinary catheter and allow about 500-800 ml of fluid at a time
- Do not clamp the irrigation tube
- Assess the color of the return flow and continue irrigation till the return flow is clear

Ear irrigation:

- Ear irrigation is done to remove discharge of the ear canal, to soften and remove impacted cerumen or to dislodge a foreign object
- Make the patient sit up or lie with the head tilted toward the side of affected ear and support a basin under the ear to receive irrigating fluid
- Wear sterile gloves
- Fill the bulb syringe with solution (warm water/NS) and check for air bubbles
- Straighten the auditory canal by pulling the pinna down and back (infant) and up and back (adult)
- Direct a steady, stream flow of solution against the roof of the auditory canal, using only sufficient force to remove secretions; do not occlude the auditory canal with the irrigating nozzle and allow solution to flow out unimpeded
- Continue to irrigate till the ear is clear of discharge
- Dry the ear with sterile cotton applicator
- When the irrigation is completed, place a dry cotton ball loosely in the auditory meatus and have the patient lie on the side of the affected ear on a towel/underpad
- Precautions:
  - o Avoid dropping or squirting on the TM
  - o Never use >500 ml of solution
  - o Monitor temperature of the solution
  - o Forceful instillation of the solution can rupture TM
  - o If pain/dizziness occurs, stop
- If irrigation is done to dislodge the wax, it is better to soften it by putting soda glycerin or H_2O_2 3-4 days prior to the procedure
- If syringe is used, do not use a large syringe as it is difficult to control and may exert undue pressure in forcing the fluid into the auditory canal

Eye irrigation:

- Eyes are flushed with solution to remove secretion and foreign bodies
- Make the patient sit up or lie with the head tilted toward the side of affected eye
- Wear sterile gloves
- Clean the lids and the lashes with a cotton ball moistened with normal saline (or other solution); wipe from the inner canthus to the outer canthus and discard the cotton ball after each wipe
- Place the curved basin at the cheek on the affected side to receive the irrigating fluid; if sitting up, patient can hold the basin
- Expose the lower conjunctival sac and hold the upper lid open with non-dominant hand
- Hold the irrigator about 2.5 cm from the eye; direct the flow of the solution from the inner canthus to the outer canthus along the conjunctival sac
- Irrigate until the solution is clear or all solution has been used; use only sufficient force gently to remove secretions from the conjunctiva; avoid touching any part of the irrigating tip
- Make the patient close the eye periodically during the procedure
- Dry the area after the irrigation with cotton balls or a gauze sponge
- For chemical burns, irrigate each eye with at least 1L of NS and irrigation could last for 10-15 minutes

BLOOD TRANSFUSION

Blood transfusion:

- Purpose:
  - o To treat severe anemia or thrombocytopenia
  - o To treat critically ill patient (massive blood loss, major surgery etc.)
  - o To provide selected cellular components as a replacement therapy (clotting factors, platelets)
- Confirm the blood grouping and typing and cross matching details (to prevent incorrect blood component transfusion error)
- Check patient vital signs (pulse, BP, respiration and temperature)
- Check the following details in blood component:
  - o Blood group and cross match
  - o Donor's and patient's name
  - o Date of blood drawn and expiry
  - o Check for any clots or any other abnormality, if found, the blood/blood product is returned to blood bank
- I/V cannula is checked for the patency before the BT is started
- Check for the patient's vital signs every 15 minutes during the first hour, followed by every 30 minutes till the BT is completed
- This helps to identify any abnormalities (allergic reaction) in early stages
- Finish the BT within 4 hours
- If any reaction occurs:
  - o Stop BT
  - o Give I/V Avil and Dexona
  - o Remaining blood is sent back to blood bank

ENEMA AND SUPPOSITORY

Types of enema:

- Evacuant:
  - o Simple
  - o Medicated
  - o Cold
- Retained:
  - o Stimulant
  - o Nutrient
  - o Emollient
  - o Sedative
  - o Anesthetic

Insertion of enema:

- Enema is the process of instilling fluid through the anal sphincter into the rectum and lower intestine
- This is done to stimulate peristalsis and to evacuate stool from the rectum
- Procedure: Explain the procedure to the patient and its importance
- Wash the hands and wear the gloves, apron and mask
- Collect history of any previous anorectal surgery or abnormalities
- Adjust the I/V stand height to hang the enema can at the required height
- Connect all the tubing and clamp in the enema can and hung the can in I/V stand
- Place the mackintosh under the patient
- Position the patient on the bed on lateral decubitus with the top knee bent and pulsed slightly upward towards the chin
- Allow the small amount of the fluid to run into the kidney tray by releasing the clamp
- Apply the lubricant jelly in the distal part of the enema tube (3-4 inch)
- Ask the patient to take deep breath and advance the tube 3-4 inches into the rectal area
- Release the clamp and allow the solution to go inside
- Solution should be in room temperature
- Ensure the prescribed amount of fluid has passed, once it does, clamp the tube
- Gently remove the tube by using the adequate gauze pieces and hold the patient's buttocks together

- Instruct the patient to hold the fluid for 5-10 minutes, until there is a strong urge to defecate
- If the patient wants to pass motion immediately, give bedpan or assess the patient to the toilet

Depth of insertion of tube:

- Adults: 3.5 to 4 inches
- Child: 2.5 to 3 inches
- Infants: Up to 1.5 inches

Suppository administration:

- Insert suppositories about 4 cm into the rectum usually using the index finger
- After procedure clean the patient perianal area and ask the patient to retain the suppository
- A suppository usually takes 20 minutes to dissolve
- Ensure that assistance is available if the patient is unable to walk to the toilet

SUTURING

Suturing techniques:

- Interrupted sutures:
  - o Simple S
  - o Mattress S
- Continuous sutures:
  - o Simple
  - o Locked/blanket
  - o Purse string

Interrupted S:

- Useful for skin closure
- Given when we anticipate serous or blood collection w/i the wound, since the gap between the stitches drains the collection
- Also, in case of infection, it is possible with interrupted stitches to remove one of the stitches

Simple interrupted S:

- Most commonly used sutures for wound closure
- But inversion of the skin edges takes place, so they are not preferable
- The knots are tied with reef knots

Mattress S:

- With this, we get eversion of skin edges
- Excessive use of force leads to devitalization of the skin or cutting through

Continuous S:

- Can be carried out rapidly to achieve good wound closure and have fewer knots
- In case of serous/blood collection, one has to remove the entire stitch, since fluid cannot escape through this type of stitch

Simple continuous S:

- This is used to close the peritoneum, rectus sheath and intestinal anastomosis

Locked/Blanket:

- Used to approximate skin edges

Purse string:

- Useful to bury the stump of the appendix into the cecal wall
- In case of skin closure where stitches must be removed, we use NA sutures
- If we wish to leave the sutures, use absorbable S

Removal of sutures:

- Usually sutures are removed between 7th - 10th day
- Knot held with thumb forceps and suture cut with scissor of surgical knife
- Clean the area with spirit

TRAUMATIC WOUND DRESSING

Traumatic wound dressing:

- Dress the wound with betadine solution and hydrogen peroxide
- Thorough wash with NS

- Once the wound is cleaned thoroughly, suture the wound (if it is healthy)
- Apply betadine ointment and put sterile gauzes to cover
- Apply bandage/micropore (depending upon site)

VENESECTION

Venesection:

- Cutting of the vein in order to push large amount of fluid
- Especially in shock patients, particularly hypovolemic shock due to loss of large amount of fluid/blood and in burn
- C/I:
  - o Varicose veins
  - o Thrombophlebitis
  - o DVT
- Common site:
  - o Long saphenous vein, 1.25 cm above and in front of medial malleolus
- Procedure: Keep the drip set ready
- Clean the part with savlon and spirit
- Drape the parts by sterile towel
- Inject 2 ml of lignocaine at the site in the S/C tissue to produce a wheal of 2 cm in diameter
- Now make a transverse incision 1.5 cm long at the selected site across the vein
- The skin is cut and the vein in S/C tissue is dissected with artery forceps
- Vein can be easily identified by its bluish tinge
- Now a curved artery forceps is passed behind the vein and with its help, two threads are passed behind the vein
- Distal one is tied and V incision is put over the vein with the help of sharp pointed scissors
- The flap is raised and a suitable cannula is passed into the vein
- On the outer end of the cannula, a proper fitting needle and drip set is attached
- Then the drip is started
- If the infusion goes smoothly, then the proximal ligature fixing the cannula is tied
- A sterile dressing is applied
- Maximum time for which venesection can be used is 72 hours
- Thereafter the site should be changed

NEEDLE-STICK INJURY

Post needlestick injury protocol:

- All health care professionals are at risk
- Exposure to blood, semen, vaginal secretions, CSF, peritoneal, pleural and pericardial fluid, amniotic fluid and other body fluids contaminated with visible blood can lead to infection
- Risk of acquiring HIV infection following percutaneous needle stick injury and after mucous membrane exposure has been estimated to be 0.3%
- Risk of HBV infection:
  - o HBeAg –ve: 6%
  - o HBeAg +ve: 40%
- Risk of HCV: 2%

Immediate care for skin:

- If the skin is broken after a needle stick injury or sharp instrument
- Immediately wash the wound and surrounding skin with water, soap and rinse
- Do not scrub
- Do not use antiseptic or skin washes (bleach, chlorine, alcohol, betadine)

Immediate care for the eye:

- Irrigate exposed eye immediately with water or NS
- Sit in a chair, tilt back and ask a colleague to gently pour water or NS over the eye

Immediate care for mouth:

- Spit fluid immediately
- Rinse the mouth thoroughly, using water or saline and spit again
- Repeat this process several times

Don nots:

- Don't panic
- Do not put pricked finger in mouth
- Do not squeeze wound to bleed
- Do not use bleach, chlorine, alcohol, betadine iodine or any other antiseptic or detergent

Standard precautions:

- Wash hands after patient contact and after removing gloves
- Wash hands immediately, if hands are contaminated with body fluids
- Wear gloves when contamination of hands with body substances is anticipated
- Protective eyewear and masks should be worn when splashing with body substances is anticipated
- Take precautions to prevent injuries during procedures and when cleaning or during disposal of needles or other sharp instruments
- Needles should not be recapped
- Needle should be purposely bent or broken by hand and not removed from disposable syringes nor manipulated by hand
- After using disposable syringes and needles, scalpel blades and other sharp instruments, they should be placed in a puncture resistant container
- Clean and disinfect blood/body substances spills with appropriate agent

SCORES

GCS:

- **E**ye opening response:
  - o Spontaneously: 4
  - o To speech: 3
  - o To pain: 2
  - o No response: 1
- Best **V**erbal response:
  - o Oriented to time, place and person: 5
  - o Confused: 4
  - o Inappropriate words: 3
  - o Incomprehensible sounds: 2
  - o No response: 1
- Best **M**otor response:
  - o Obeys commands: 6
  - o Moves to localized pain: 5
  - o Flexion withdrawal from pain: 4
  - o Abnormal flexion (decorticate): 3
  - o Abnormal extension (decerebrate): 2
  - o No response: 1
- Total score:
  - o Best response: 15
  - o Comatose client: 8 or less
  - o Totally unresponsive: 3

Apgar score:

- **A**ppearance:
  - o Blue, pale skin: 0
  - o Body pink, extremities blue: 1
  - o Completely pink: 2
- **P**ulse:
  - o Absent: 0
  - o Below 100/minute: 1
  - o Above 100/minute: 2
- **G**rimace:
  - o No response: 0
  - o Grimaces: 1
  - o Cries: 2
- **A**ctivity:
  - o Limp: 0
  - o Some flexion of extremities: 1
  - o Active motion: 2
- **R**espiratory effort:
  - o Absent: 0
  - o Slow and irregular: 1
  - o Strong cry: 2
- Interpretation of score:
  - o 0-3:
    - Severely depressed neonate

  - Needs resuscitation: CPR, intubation, ventilate with 100% oxygen, maintain body temperature
- o 4-6:
  - Moderately depressed neonate
  - Airway clearance
  - Suction immediately
- o 7-10:
  - Good adjustment
  - Routine newborn care

CONDITIONS AND PREFERRED POSITIONS

Conditions and preferred positions of patient:

- Gynecological and abdominal hernia surgeries: Trendelenburg position
- Placement of central lines: Trendelenburg position
- Treating venous air embolism: Reverse Trendelenburg position
- Preventing pulmonary aspiration: Reverse Trendelenburg position
- Administering enemas: Sim's position
- Perineal examination: Sim's position
- Drainage of mouth after oral/neck surgeries: Prone position
- Gynecological procedures: Lithotomy position
- Cardiac issues: Fowler's position
- Nasogastric tube in place: Fowler's position
- Breathing difficulty: Fowler's position